BY EMILY NAGOSKI, PhD

Come Together:
The Science (and Art!) of Creating Lasting
Sexual Connections

Come as You Are:
The Surprising New Science That
Will Transform Your Sex Life

Burnout:
The Secret to Unlocking the Stress Cycle,
with Amelia Nagoski

Come Together

Come Together

Together

THE SCIENCE (AND ART!)
OF CREATING LASTING
SEXUAL CONNECTIONS

EMILY NAGOSKI, PhD

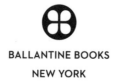

BALLANTINE BOOKS

NEW YORK

Published in the United States by Ballantine Books, an imprint of Random House, a division of Penguin Random House LLC, New York.

BALLANTINE BOOKS & colophon are registered trademarks of Penguin Random House LLC.

Library of Congress Cataloging-in-Publication Data
Names: Nagoski, Emily, author.
Title: Come together: the science (and art!) of creating lasting sexual connections / Emily Nagoski.
Description: New York: Ballantine Books, [2024] | Includes bibliographical references and index.
Identifiers: LCCN 2023028256 (print) | LCCN 2023028257 (ebook) | ISBN 9780593500828 (hardcover) | ISBN 9780593500842 (ebook)
Subjects: LCSH: Sexual excitement. | Sex (Psychology) | Interpersonal relations.
Classification: LCC HQ31 .N247 2024 (print) | LCC HQ31 (ebook) | DDC 155.3/1—dc23/eng/20230802
LC record available at https://lccn.loc.gov/2023028256
LC ebook record available at https://lccn.loc.gov/2023028257

Printed in the United States of America on acid-free paper

randomhousebooks.com

2 4 6 8 9 7 5 3 1

Book design by Alexis Capitini
First Edition

For rstevens,
the marital euphemism

CONTENTS

INTRODUCTION

"How Do I Fix It?"

Once upon a time (around 2014) I wrote *Come as You Are*, a book about the science of women's sexual well-being. Ironically, the process of thinking, reading, and writing every day about sex made me so stressed that I had zero interest in actually *having* any sex.

For months, nothing.

My partner was incredibly patient and understanding, even as I felt guilty.

Then the book was published! I went on a book tour! I traveled all over, talking to anyone who would listen about the science of women's sexual well-being! And when I got home from these trips, I'd try to connect sexually with my partner, but most of the time I'd get into the bed and . . . just fall asleep.

More months! Of *nothing*!!

It went on for so long that eventually I became distanced from my partner and from my own erotic self, knocked down and carried away by the fatigue, overwhelm, health issues, and existential crises that seemed to come at me in wave after wave of anti-erotic daily life.

I missed sex. I missed that connection with my partner, and I missed the part of myself that plays in the erotic realm.

I am the kind of person who would like to continue developing a sexual connection with my certain special someone far into our old age. I want to be giggling and licking and snuggling when we're ninety-five, if we're lucky enough to live so long.

And I'm far from alone—which is why there are so many books and articles and general advice for couples who want to know how to have a happy sex life in a long-term relationship. Most of us struggle at some point to maintain that connection, and we're looking for solutions.

As a science-loving sex educator, I had a nerdy approach when it came to solving my own sexual difficulties: I went right to the peer-reviewed research. What I found there contradicted all the widespread (but false!) narratives about "keeping the spark alive." You may have an image in your mind of what a great long-term sexual relationship is like—what kind of sex those people have, how often they have it, where and when they do it, and what it feels like when they have it.

It turns out, probably all of those things are wrong.

What do you think is the key to great sex over the long term?

Some people think it's about frequency. It's not.[1] There's very little relationship between frequency of sex and sexual or relationship satisfaction. Hardly any of us has sex very often; *we are busy.*

Some people think it's novelty and adventure. It's not. And it's not orgasms, sex positions, variety of sexual behaviors, or anything else. Honestly? If there's a "sexual behavior" that predicts sex and relationship satisfaction, it's cuddling after sex.[2] Wildly original sex might be enjoyable for you (or it might not), but it is not what makes for a satisfying long-term sex life for most people.

People think the key to satisfying long-term sex is monogamy or nonmonogamy; watching porn or not watching porn; being kinky or vanilla.[3] It's not. Those are all just different ways people engage sexually and emotionally with the world, and whether they work for you or not is a matter of personal experience. People can have great (or terrible) sex lives either way.

People think it's attractiveness, being conventionally good-looking, or it's having a perfect relationship or a perfect body, or it's "skills" like knowing a lot about how to give great oral sex. None of those things predict great sex in the long-term. The idea of a "skilled" lover is a myth; unless you're trying technically demanding BDSM practice like breath play, the only "skill" you need is the ability to pay attention to your partner and to your own internal experience at the same time.[4]

Perhaps above all, people think it's an out-of-the-blue craving for sex, the hot-and-heavy horny feeling that makes people constantly want to put their tongues in each other's mouths. This is often what people mean when they talk about "the spark" that we're all supposed to want to keep alive.

The science taught me three essential characteristics of couples who sustain a connection over the long term, and none of them were the characteristics you might guess.

I'm happy to give away the ending right here at the start. The three characteristics of partnerships that sustain a strong sexual connection are:

1. They are friends—or, to put it more precisely, they trust and admire each other.

2. They prioritize sex—that is, they decide that it matters for their relationship.

3. Instead of accepting other people's opinions about how they're supposed to do sex in their partnership, they prioritize what's genuinely true for them and what works in their unique relationship.

And what do they do, these friends who prioritize sex and prioritize each other over any prefabricated notions of what sex is supposed to be?

They co-create a context that makes it easier to access pleasure. That's it.

Once I saw the pattern, it felt so liberating, so forgiving, so darn *doable* that I wanted to share it with everyone.

So I wrote this book, to explain this surprisingly simple truth about sex in long-term relationships and to provide concrete, specific tools for maximizing the erotic potential in any happy long-term sexual connection.

This book represents my decades of experience as a sex educator, a decade of advancement in the research literature, and a decade of marriage in which my own sexual connection with my partner ebbed and flowed.

You might be in a monogamous partnership or you might be in an open relationship, or you might be in a committed thruple, multuple (I think I made that word up, but it sounds right, right?), or polycule. Maybe you were in a long-term relationship in which the sexual connection didn't last, and you'd like to understand why that happened and how to prevent it in the future. Maybe you haven't yet been in a long-term relationship but you would like to be someday, and you want to know how to build a sexual connection, from day one, that will last. If you're a human who lives in a body and wants to know more about having good sex, really good sex, spectacular sex, and universe-dissolving sex with another person over the long term, this book is for you.

The promise of *Come Together* is this: You will learn what great sex over the long term looks like in real life, how to create it in your own life, and what to do when struggles arise—which they definitely will.

How to Use This Book

My quarter of a century as a sex educator has taught me that people crave simple, step-by-step instructions to help them get from where they are to where they want to be, presented in a series of well-defined, predictable stages. Sometimes people pick up a book like this, already impatient for answers about their specific situation; they want me to just *explain what to do*!!!

"Just fix it!" they shout at the book.

I felt that way. I was shouting it at *myself.*

But.

I can't tell you how to "fix" your sexuality . . . because you are not broken.

Instead of thinking about your sexuality as a problem that needs to be fixed, think of it in terms of the garden metaphor I used throughout *Come as You Are* (*CAYA*):

On the day you are born, you are given a brand-new field of rich and fertile soil—the garden of your sexuality. And immediately, your family begins to plant ideas about bodies and gender and sex and pleasure and safety and love. Your culture enters with various weeds and invasive species—windblown seeds of myths about the "ideal sexual person" and ropes of vines about beauty standards, spreading like poison ivy under the fence and over the garden wall.

Some of us get lucky. Our families weeded out the invaders and only planted healthy, pleasure-forward ideas, and so all we have to do is tend and harvest.

Most of us, though, get stuck with some pretty toxic crap. We're left with the task of going through our gardens row by row, examining what we find there, and making choices about what to keep and cultivate . . . and what to pull and throw on the compost heap to rot.

It is not fair that we have to do this work. After all, we didn't get to choose any of the plants our families and cultures planted in our gardens. No one waited until we could give consent and asked, "Would it be okay if I planted this giant, suffocating vine of shame right here?" No, they just let it grow—sometimes even fertilized it with their own shame.

It's not fair that we have these toxic things in our gardens; we never chose them. But it is an *opportunity*. It is your chance to create a sexual mind that *you choose for yourself,* instead of one inherited from a family or a culture that offered you little opportunity to express an opinion about what worked for your growing garden.

Your sexuality is not a problem you have to solve or a disorder that needs to be treated. Your sexuality is a garden you can cultivate.

What I didn't mention in *CAYA* is what happens when you decide to co-create a shared garden with someone else, with the idea that you'll continue to tend this garden for many years to come.

You each bring plants from your individual gardens and help propagate plants from your partner's garden, too, finding ways to arrange them so that every plant has what it needs to thrive. Because you plan to have years together, you have plenty of time; you can experiment and, if things don't go as planned, you have opportunities to repair any damage you might inadvertently do.

A shared garden may be started with enthusiasm, but then at some point, the mismatch of the gardens you're transplanting may feel insurmountable and so you give up. Or changes in the relationship don't provide a good enough environment for the garden to thrive. Or, other priorities take over and the garden is neglected. It happens. It happened to me.

With time, we can get better and better at cultivating the garden, maximizing its beauty, its bounty, learning from the garden itself how best to tend it. Over years, you learn its cycles, from the barrenness of short, cold days to the abundance of the long, warm days.

When you do the work of cultivating your individual garden and your shared garden, you're not just doing good for yourself and your erotic relationship, you're doing good *for the world*. Every time you pull the invasive weeds of body self-criticism or sexual shame, you weaken the social vine, making it that much easier for your sister to pull it from her garden, or your daughter or your niece, your clients and patients, your romantic and sexual partners. When you cultivate a garden that is uniquely your own, filled with whatever brings you delight, you make it a little easier for everyone else to do the same.

How the Book Is Organized

Come Together is organized into two parts:

In the first part of the book, "Pleasure Is the Measure," I'll describe how couples can sustain a strong sexual connection over the long term. I'll talk about what matters in a sexual connection, what it means to prioritize sex, what happens in our brains to facilitate or inhibit sexual interest, and what to do about it. I'll also describe essential tools for creating a context that makes it easier to access pleasure.

In the second part, "Good Things Come," I apply all those tools to the issues that often arise in long-term sexual relationships, including both relationship difficulties and cultural barriers. My goal in part 2 is to provide you with practical guidance for building and maintaining a lasting sexual connection. What no one ever told me, and what I want to make sure we all know, is that urgency is the enemy of pleasure. Even as we acknowledge that we don't know what the future holds, we can approach changes to our sexual relationships as if we have plenty of time.

As in *Come as You Are* and *Burnout,* you'll follow the stories of a number of composite characters. These are real stories that I've blended together to create examples of how different kinds of partners can apply the information in this book to their actual relationships. Mike and Kendra, Ama and Di, and Margot and Hugh are not specific individuals I know, but their stories are made from the stories of people I know. I use composites like this to show not just individual moments in a couple's life but a whole arc of how partners can process and change and grow together over time.

In appendix 1 you'll find what I call the "But, Emily!" questions—the kind of questions I get from people who may have learned the science but haven't yet found a way to integrate it into their lives. Questions like "But, Emily, what if the problem is actually just my partner?" or "But, Emily, I just want my partner to want me so much they can't help themselves! How do I make that happen?" My responses there will direct you to the specific places in this book (or in other books) that can help you find your way to your own answers.

In the end, you'll have the knowledge and skills to maximize the erotic potential between yourself and a long-term partner. And maybe most important: You'll see the vast potential, the enormous opportunity available to us all, when we decide to co-create a garden with someone through many seasons, over many years.

A Caveat about Science

I love science. It's a powerful antidote to the false moralistic messages so many of us grow up with around sex. So I rely on it in this and in all of my books. But science is not the only way to learn about the world, and, like all ways of knowing, it has its limits. I put a science caveat in all my books, but it's even more important here than in the others:

Science is done by people, and people are products of their time. In my search for research that included a wide variety of people, I spent more time sifting through biased, noninclusive papers than reading good stuff. It's not just that research on "women's sexuality" is almost exclusively about cisgender women, it's also that a study that includes 90 percent or more white women participants is described as a study of *all* women's sexuality, rather than of white women's sexuality. A study of autistic people's sexuality compares people on the spectrum to "healthy controls," and that got published in the late 2010s as if it wasn't grotesquely problematic. (Autistic people are not "diseased," please and thank you.) Polyamorous and monogamous relationships are very often studied separately, as if human connection is somehow fundamentally different, depending on relationship structure. Transgender people participate in sex research, and the researchers write about the results in language that would almost certainly feel deeply offensive to the trans participants. I'm not including endnotes for any of those examples because I don't think they need to be read by anyone. Until the science is better, I can't write an inclusive book that's closely and transparently linked to the research. Because *Come Together* is for everyone interested in sex in a long-term relationship, this book relies as much on conversations with actual people, who are the true experts of their own experience, as it does on academic research.

Another caveat—the kind of caveat more science should address: I write from a specific social location that involves a whole bunch of privilege. I'm a white, cisgender woman from the northeastern United States, with three academic degrees. I'm not straight, but I benefit from straight privilege. My disabilities are largely invisible, so I benefit from able-bodied privilege. My age and my body shape are always changing, like everyone else's, but currently I'm smack-dab in the middle of the middle—Gen X and "small fat."[5]

Despite the limitations inherent in my social location, my goal is for every reader to find themselves in this book, so I've included stories and research from people very different from me, including people of different races, religions, ethnicities, genders, sexual orientations, and sexual or romantic relationship structures; people with different experiences of childhood and parenthood, different experiences of formal education and neurodivergence, and people with differently shaped bodies, different ages, different physical abilities, and different mental health experiences. I hope I've done their stories justice.

So. Deep cleansing breaths. Get ready to take a little time to explore your gardens and figure out what they need.

Begin the first page of chapter 1 by reminding yourself: *I'm not broken.* No one is broken. We are all doing our best with the imperfect resources available to us in this imperfect world.

Just as a long-neglected garden can be tended and brought to new life and glory, an erotic garden can bloom again. This book has already done that for me. It can do the same for you.

PART 1

Pleasure Is the Measure

Chapter 1

IS SEX IMPORTANT?

In this first part of the book, I'm introducing a different way to think about sex: What if we shelve the entire concept of desire and, in its place, prioritize *pleasure* and how we create it in our lives? If you enjoy the sex you're having, you're doing great, regardless of how much you crave sex (or don't) and regardless of how often you have it (or don't).

Great sex in a long-term relationship is not about how much you desire sex or how often you have to do it. It's not about what you do, in which position, with whom or where or in what clothes, even how many orgasms you have. It's whether or not you like the sex you are having.

Your task, as a partnership, is to explore ways to co-create a shared context—a shared life, a connection, a state of mind, a way of being together—that makes pleasure easy to access. It starts with understanding why sex matters in your relationship—if it matters, which it doesn't always. It continues with considering when and why and how sex feels good—if it feels good, which it doesn't always.

So how important *is* sex?

¯_(ツ)_/¯

Sex is really important to some people, in some relationships or in some specific contexts. But in terms of getting through our day-to-day lives, sex is generally no big deal. Nobody's going to die or even get sick if they don't have sex.[1] Nobody is diseased or dysfunctional if sex seems like more trouble than it's worth, just as nobody is diseased or dysfunctional if sex feels urgently important, day after day.

Regardless of whether sex seems important or not, there are only twenty-four hours in a day and seven days in a week. Nobody gets more, and we have a lot of things to do in that time. Maybe we have family to take care of, maybe we have a paycheck to earn, an academic degree to finish, chores to do, a puppy to house-train, a chronic illness to manage. We have to sleep, eat, bathe, maybe talk to friends who are not our sex partners, maybe even, god forbid, we just want to watch a little TV and take a nap.

When my own sex life evaporated, I had an advantage most people don't: I knew that the couples who sustain a satisfying sexual connection are the couples who decide that sex matters enough for their relationship that they cordon off space, time, and energy specifically for sex. They stop doing all those other things they could be doing, they close the door on all those other responsibilities and enjoyments, and they turn toward each other's erotic selves.

But why, when we have so many other things we could be doing, do we choose to have sex?

Why Have Sex?

Let's face it, sex is kind of silly. We dignified humans put our tongues in each other's mouths, we put our mouths on each other's genitals, we rub our skins together and wrestle like puppies, we let our bodies roll through orgasm even when there's someone else there to witness it. We bounce and grunt and spasm and ooze. What in the world is happening in the midst of all that silliness that makes it worth stopping everything else just to do *that*?

For some of you, it's a no-brainer. You can't even understand why it's a question. If you're one of the people for whom sex is very, very important—and maybe just reading that "sex is only important sometimes to some people" makes you a little panicky—never fear. You are normal! But even you won't die or be injured or get sick if you don't do this silly, often delightful, sometimes not at all good, occasionally extremely important thing we humans can do.

For some of you, "Why have sex?" is a question you've been asking yourself privately for years. You may feel kind of relieved or even vindicated to read that sex doesn't have to be very important. And you're normal, too!

Regardless of how you feel about the idea that sex doesn't have to be a big deal, here's a question that I want you to consider very seriously:

What is it that you want when you want sex with a partner?

Hint: The answer is generally not "an orgasm." If you want an orgasm, have an orgasm.[2] You can do that on your own. But what is it that you want when you want to have sex with the partner with whom you plan to sustain a sexual connection for the foreseeable future?

Take your time with this and go deep. What is it about sex *with this other person* that motivates and inspires you? What is your partner giving you when they give you their erotic attention? What do you receive when you receive their touch? And if some part of you is thinking, *I just want sex, and this is the only person I'm supposed to be having it with soooooooo . . .* consider what it is about sex with another person that matters. What changes when there's someone else there for you to touch and be touched by?

Over the last several years, I've asked a few hundred people this question. At workshops, during online events, and in internet surveys, I've asked people to let me know their answers to this question, to give me a better sense of what images and priorities pop up in their minds.[3]

In my informal surveys, the answers to the question "What do you want when you want sex with a partner?" usually came down to what I've started to call The Big Four: Connection, Shared Pleasure, Being Wanted, and Freedom.

1. CONNECTION. Overwhelmingly, the most common thing people reported wanting is connection with their partner. What precisely do people mean by connection? I'll leave that to you to define. But some of the responses I received show that "connection" can be physical and emotional and more than both—e.g.,

> "I want to hold and be held and make out and explore each other's bodies."

> "I want to feel listened to and taken care of."

If "connection" is part of your own answer, you can ask yourself further questions like: What does connection feel like? Where in my body, mind, and/or spirit do I experience connection? What words or behaviors increase my sense of connection?

2. SHARED PLEASURE. Like orgasm, pleasure is something we can experience on our own, but that is not what people say they want when they want sex with a partner. Most often, it's the pleasure of witnessing a partner's pleasure, experiencing our partner's enjoyment of our own pleasure, or *sharing* pleasure. People do not just want to enjoy the sensation of rubbing body parts against someone else; we want pleasure for everyone involved. People said things like:

> "I want someone caring about my pleasure."

> "I want to focus on my partner's body—her movements and tastes and sounds and smells."

Our partners' pleasure matters to us, and we want our own pleasure to matter to our partners.

3. BEING WANTED. This was about as commonly mentioned as pleasure. What people want when they want sex is *to be wanted* by their partner; not just in response to pleasure we co-create, but in anticipation of the pleasure we can share:

> *"I want to feel like my partner loves and appreciates every aspect of my body and mind, even the flaws."*

> *"I want approval and acceptance."*

Others described it as wanting "to feel desirable" or "to feel sexy." When I spoke with people for whom feeling desired or desirable was what they wanted, a lot of what they wanted, underneath the experience of being desired, was validation. Many of us are carrying around hurt parts of ourselves that are, on some level, convinced we are undesirable or even unlovable, and being desired soothes that part of ourselves.

A perimenopausal queer woman, reflecting on the casual sex of her twenties, put it this way: "There are parts of me that fundamentally believe I am unfuckable and those are the parts of me that wanted to feel desired. There was a physical craving, and it was exciting, but [sex] met the needs of the parts of me that need to be desired."

If something you want, when you want sex with a partner, is to feel sexy/desirable or to be or feel desired, try asking the further questions: What is it that I want when I want to feel sexy or desirable? Is there something different about "desirability" versus feeling or being desired?

4. FREEDOM. This is the feeling of being fully immersed in an erotic experience. People want a feeling of *escape* from the ordinary day-to-day of their lives and a sense that they can stop thinking about anything else and experience a moment full of pleasure. They want to disappear into lust—e.g.,

"I want to clear my head and stop thinking. To be so into my partner that the world falls away."

"I want to relax and relinquish control and be completely present."

The opposite emerged, too, when respondents described what they *didn't* want or like. People don't want or like sex when they feel distracted, their minds pulled in a million directions. They don't want or like pressure to "perform." They don't want or like feeling obligated to have sex.

In short, when people want sex, often what they want is to be free from wanting anything else. They want to step away from stressors, suffering, dissatisfaction, and distress. They want to step into a space too full of pleasure for there to be room for anything else.

"I Don't Want It"

It's important to note that some people just don't want sex, even if they want the other things that can come with sex. They say things like:

"I can't even remember the last time I really wanted sex."

"I don't really want it, in general. I think when I did want it—in the past—what I really wanted was approval, not sex."

If that's you, hi, hello! You are not required to want sex! You are allowed to have your needs and desires met through experiences that are not sexual.

There are many ways a person can come to not want sex. Maybe they're asexual (ace)—that is, they don't experience sexual attraction to anyone, even when they may be romantically or aesthetically attracted to people. Or maybe they've experienced a lot of disappointing, painful, or unwanted sex, and now their body and mind have learned that sex is not worth wanting. Maybe they experience sexual attraction and have had great sex in the past, but they're overwhelmingly stressed, depressed, anxious, frustrated, or exhausted. It's perfectly reasonable not to want sex if the rest of your life doesn't have space for rest, pleasure, and joy.

In every case, a great next step is to grant yourself or your partner the permission *not to have to try* to want sex. For ace folks, permission not to have to try is a release from cultural narratives of "compulsory sexuality" that make people feel like failures if they don't want, like, or have lots of sex. What if you never had to try again?[4] Free! Forever!

For folks who have had a lot of bad experiences, you can enjoy not having to try to want sex while creating a context where you can heal from the bad or unwanted sex (in chapter 5 I'll talk about the woundedness to healing cycle; and in chapter 7 I'll directly address trauma, neglect, and abuse). Try connecting with pleasures of all kinds, beginning with the nonsexual—the pleasures of a breeze on your face, your favorite scent, a bite of delicious food, or watching your best friend laugh.

For the person who is overwhelmed and exhausted, the opportunity not to have to try to want sex shifts the focus from "How can I/my partner want sex more?" to "How can we help me/my partner get access to more rest and more help?"

There were a lot of pain stories in people's "I don't want sex" answers. Histories of painful yeast infections, physical and mental changes experienced with menopause, and various experiences of trauma. All of these and more were associated with not wanting or liking sex, especially when a partner seemed oblivious to the need to create space and gentleness around these histories. But perhaps most of all, stories of obligation showed up in answers about what people don't want or like, as in *"Feeling obligated, feeling like I'm performing,"* and *"Feeling uncomfortable but obligated,"* and *"Feeling like my partner is only concerned with their own orgasm, when it feels obligatory."*

So if I spend a lot of time in this book granting people permission to stop trying to have, want, or like sex, it's to help liberate readers from any sense of obligation, and to help their partners recognize the necessity of creating a space where there is no pressure, expectation, or obligation, and everyone is a little freer to explore pleasure in a context of safety and autonomy.

It's nice to quietly consider your answers to any or all of these questions on your own, but I encourage you to talk to a partner, if you have one, or a friend or therapist. The variety of what people want when they want sex with a partner is virtually infinite. I don't know what you want when you want sex with a partner, but I invite you to consider the question.

Your answers will probably change over time, as your context changes. Write down your answers now and come back to them next year or in five years or in twenty and see how you feel about what you wrote.

Margot and Henry

Henry is the Ted Lasso of polyamorous eroticism, relentlessly optimistic, a believer in belief itself, confident that hope alone can do anything. He's been married to one person since the '80s, and their marriage has always been open to other partners—sexually, emotionally, and otherwise—by mutual loving and enthusiastic consent.

I want to tell you not about Henry's relationship with his wife (who is a spectacular human with many stories of her own), but his relationship with a longtime non-householding partner, Margot. By "longtime," I mean two decades. He's been lovers with Margot for longer than I've known my husband.

Henry and Margot met when Margot was fresh out of a painful divorce. In the beginning, she loved being "secondary," a partner to someone who already had someone else to meet all their pragmatic needs, someone else to raise the kids and do the chores, and she could just enjoy time with him.

The longer they were together, the more entwined they became in each other's lives . . . and so gradually Margot became not so much a secondary partner as an additional partner. She helped take care of his kids and grandkids, and he helped take care of her kids and grandkids. (Only some of the kids were aware of their sexual connection, and none of the grandkids were. Different people make different choices around disclosing nonmonogamous relationships to their offspring.)

Because they didn't share a household, their erotic connection mostly took the form of rare, special weekends, cordoned off from other responsibilities. They would often drive a couple of hours to a gorgeous resort, to get literally geographically away from it all, for a weekend of restorative, healing, delicious, joyful pleasure. You might imagine that that would automatically create a context where it would be easy to want and like sex.

And you'd be wrong.

At the point when their story begins, Margot's life had gotten really complicated, with one of her adult children in the midst of a divorce while parenting a child with special needs. Margot was providing childcare as well as emotional support, and preparing for the possibility that her son and grandchild might be moving in with her. It was a lot.

Even under easy circumstances, in open relationships it takes a lot of people's love, generosity, time, and collaboration to create a context where a pair of people can go away for two nights, and Margot felt grateful to Henry's primary partner; to her own primary, who had taken on many family responsibilities; and to everyone else who was helping to make this weekend of peace possible . . . It's surprising how burdensome gratitude can become when so many people are being so helpful and yet you can't find your way to the peace and pleasure they're trying to facilitate.

Not only did Margot bring all her stress and worry with her to the gorgeous resort, she added to it her guilt and distress about not being able to let go of all that stuff and just focus on Henry during the special time everyone put so much effort into creating for them. She felt like she owed it not just to Henry but to herself and to all the people who were holding the fort while she was away.

And because they had just two nights, she felt pressured to get herself "in the mood" as soon as humanly possible. Which obviously made it impossible to feel anything but stressed.

Henry—the relentless optimist—suggested instead that they just talk about what they wanted when they wanted sex.

For Henry it was easy—"Well, of course I want the pleasure of it, our bodies all warm and rolling around in heat and wetness and throbbing. But I love when pleasure floods us together. I love seeing you turned on, I love when you can let go of everything else and just revel like a decadent hedonist, Jeremy Bentham's satisfied pig, pure pleasure, intense enough to counterbalance a lifetime of discipline. And I love that I get to go there with you. It's like going on the best imaginable vacation, and it's free and it's divine and it's raunchy and it's us. That's what makes sex matter to me. How about you?"

"Skipping lightly over the satisfied pig," Margot said, "What makes sex matter to me? Why would I spend time with you having sex instead of doing anything else? A lot of it is just being with you. You go there so easily, and I want to go with. You said you go there with me, but really you show me the way. But that just begs the question, doesn't it. Why go there, wherever 'there' is?"

"'There' is untethered pleasure," Henry supplied.

"Why go to untethered pleasure?" Margot wondered. "Honestly, I just know it's good for me. The pain in my hands and joints vanishes for minutes at a time. I feel grounded in this body that still isn't familiar to me. I feel held in human connection in a way that nothing else can

duplicate. Like we're naked in a hot air balloon and I'm twenty-three again, with all the good things that entails but none of the bad things. And when we come back to Earth, I carry some of that feeling with me for days afterward."

"That is important," Henry said.

"It is," Margot agreed. "And it does motivate me to make plans for us, to show up for us. But I can't say it makes it easier to untether from my life, or to stop feeling obligated to you and to everyone, to feel a certain way."

Don't worry, they figure that part out the next time we see them, in chapter 4.

Sidenote: There are a surprising number of Henrys in mid-century pop and folk songs. "Roll with Me, Henry," sometimes sung as "Dance with Me, Henry," but also "I'm Henry VIII, I Am," every folk ballad about John Henry, and Margot's favorite, "Oh, Henry," a ska-style bop sung by Millie Small, about a stray puppy who follows the singer home. I would be remiss in describing this model conversation, condensed for clarity, if I didn't mention that they took a break about halfway through to play this song and dance around their hotel room, alternating the pony with the hitchhiker and the swim.

I witness the wisdom of my elders, and I am in awe and I am grateful.

The Accelerator and the Brakes

By answering questions like "What is it that I want when I want sex?" you're building a sense of what makes sex worth not watching TV for. If we know *why* sex with our partner is important, if it's important, we can then focus on how to create a context to make it happen.

Your brain has opinions about when sex is (or isn't) important. This is because of a brain mechanism that will be familiar to folks who read *Come as You Are*. When you first learn about it, it feels completely revelatory, but once you know it, it feels like you always knew it. It's this:

The brain mechanism that governs sexual response has two parts, the accelerator and the brakes. The accelerator notices all the sex-related stimuli in the environment—everything you see, hear, smell, touch, taste, think, believe, or imagine, plus all your internal body sensations that it codes as relevant to sex—and it sends the "turn on" signal many of us are familiar with. It's working all the time, below conscious awareness. All kinds of things can activate the accelerator, from the sound of your partner's voice to the sight of a sexy body part or watching them do something completely non-sexual that makes you feel admiring of them and lucky to be their partner. A lot of your "What is it that I want when I want sex?" answers will be things that activate the accelerator.

The brakes notice all the good reasons not to be turned on right now—everything you see, hear, smell, touch, taste, think, believe, or imagine, plus your internal body sensations that your brain codes as a potential threat—and it sends the "turn off" signal. It, too, functions all the time, below conscious awareness. All kinds of things can hit the brakes, from relationship conflict to stress and exhaustion to trauma or body image issues to sex negative cultural messages to worry that the kids will interrupt to irritating grit on the sheets.

Your level of sexual arousal at any given moment is a balance of how much the accelerator is activated and how much the brakes are being hit.

When people are struggling with any dimension of sexual functioning, whether it's orgasm, desire, arousal, or pleasure, sometimes it's because there's not enough stimulation to the accelerator. A longtime friend of mine, married with two kids and who has extraordinary communication with her partner, thought about the question "What is it that I want when I want sex with my partner?" in a different way. She asked, "What kind of sex is worth not doing anything else?" She thought about it and said to her partner, "What

I really love is when you pull my hair like you sometimes do, especially while you fuck me from behind, you know?"

Her partner's response? "Oh! Yeah! I mean, I can do that!" Was he bothered by her bluntness? Did he feel criticized or judged? Heck no, because all he heard was praise about the things he was already doing well.

Sometimes it's that simple.

But often it's not. Often, problems exist not due to lack of stimulation to the accelerator, but because there's *too much stimulation to the brakes.* The brakes turn on because, as far as your brain is concerned, sex is not a priority right in this moment.

That means it's normal to feel less arousal, less desire, and less pleasure, when you're worried about money or the kids, when work is really stressful, when you're in the midst of an argument with your partner, when you feel like you have an obligation to have sex to satisfy your partner but actually you'd prefer to finish folding the laundry while listening to a podcast, or when sex is painful, boring, or otherwise unpleasant. Normal! Not a dysfunction! There is nothing wrong with your sexual response that a change in your *context* won't fix.

Some really good questions to ask yourself are:

- What activates the accelerator? These are the things that increase arousal, pleasure, and interest in sex.

- What hits the brakes? These are things that decrease arousal, pleasure, and interest in sex.

- How can you create a context that activates the accelerator more and, even better, hits the brakes less?

Feel free to write lists of things that, off the top of your head, you know hit your brakes or activate the accelerator.

I have been asking people to write these lists for more than a decade, in workshops and seminars. Here's a little of what they say, to kick-start your own brainstorming.

CAN ACTIVATE THE ACCELERATOR	CAN HIT THE BRAKES
• Non-sexual touch	• Pain
• Intimacy of various kinds	• Anxiety or depression (or both)
• Trust—both trusting a partner and feeling trusted by a partner	• Pressure/expectation/a sense of obligation or "duty"
• Stress—adrenaline, fight-or-flight, or loneliness	• Stress—overwhelm, depletion, frustration about anything, including about sex
• Flirtation and affectionate teasing	• Being tired/exhausted/fatigued
• Intellectual or emotionally intimate conversation	• Lack of emotional connection
• Knowing we have all the time we need	• Feeling rushed/like my partner is impatient
• Enjoying relaxed time with my partner	• Feeling manipulated or pressured to have sex
• Talking about sex	• Talking about sex
• Partner's enthusiasm/ knowing my partner wants it	• Not feeling like my partner wants it
• The excitement of potentially being "caught"	• Distractions/when thoughts intrude
• Wearing sexy clothes/ my partner wearing sexy clothes	• Worry about potentially being interrupted
• Excitement of potentially being overheard	• Worry about body image
	• Worry about people overhearing

As you can see, things that activate the accelerator for some people may hit the brakes for others. For some people, the real risk of being interrupted hits the brakes when they're having sex with their partner, but when they're solo masturbating, the fantasy of that risk can activate the accelerator.

Here's another question to ask yourself and your partner: When you think about a time when pleasure was easy, how were you feeling about your job, money, family, or the state of the world?

A lot of people, especially those who are struggling around sex, can often list lots of things that hit the brakes (the kids! work! my partner's parents! money! the news! I'm so tired!), but then they sit there, stymied, as they try to imagine what activates the accelerator. If you feel yourself getting stuck at any point, it can often help to remember a positive sexual experience or fantasy you've had and consider what it is about that experience or fantasy that works for you.

Sometimes your hypothetical ideas about what makes a great sexy context don't translate to real life the way you expect. An older gay couple I know made a New Year's resolution to have at least a little sex every day. They thought it would keep the "spark" alive, being sexually connected every twenty-four hours. At first, it did. They tried new things, explored and experimented together. But after a few weeks, they were overwhelmed by the sense that sex was a chore that they were just getting through instead of enjoying, all because they decided on this *project*. They had unwittingly created a context where they felt obligated to have sex, and feeling obligated is among the most universal of brakes-hitting contexts.

They replaced "at least a little sex every day" with "only light stuff every day, except for one day a week when we can do anything." "Light stuff" for them was mostly non-genital touching. They could kiss and pet, touch and rub, but no oral sex, manual sex, or genital-to-genital touching. That was much more fun, because the "light" days acted as a kind of weeklong foreplay for their one day of anything they liked.

Experiments like this are why the best sex advice won't come from a book. It will come from the way you use your knowledge of the accelerator and brakes and of what you each want and like about sex, and from the way you communicate with each other about all of that.

Here's one of my favorite examples: A woman, her husband, and their three kids always vacationed in the same little town on the Mediterranean Sea, renting the same ancient and beautiful house each year. And she and her husband always had *great* vacation sex. One year their usual house wasn't available, but no worries, they got a different beautiful rental. But this year . . . mediocre vacation sex! What happened?

When they got home from vacation, she and her husband thought carefully about their internal experiences in each home and came to a simple realization: Their usual vacation house was so old the bed was built into the wall! That meant no squeaking or bumping, no worrying about the kids waking up and interrupting! With that one distraction gone, they were free to enjoy themselves without part of their brains constantly monitoring for noise. The unsqueaky bed turned out to be a key to their amazing sex.

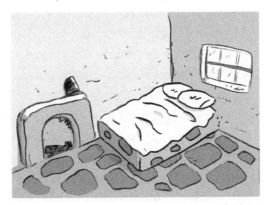

In some old houses in the Mediterranean, the beds are built into the wall.

Instead of being worried about or ashamed of the difficulty, this couple was *curious* about it, together, which turns out to be an essential tool when trying to solve a sex problem. Instead of asking, "What's wrong?" they chose to ask, "What's hitting the brakes?"

The story has a twist happy ending! When they built their own non-vacation, everyday house, they built the bed into the wall of the primary bedroom.

I would never think to advise someone to build their bed into the wall like an ancient Mediterranean house. That's a solution you find by understanding why you have sex and why, sometimes, you don't.

Chapter 1 tl;dr:

- What people want when they want sex, is not mere orgasm, but connection, pleasure, feeling wanted, and a sense of freedom from ordinary life.

- Some people, for any number of reasons, might not want sex. A great question to ask in that case is "What is it that I *don't* want, when I don't want sex?"

- Your brain has both a sexual accelerator, which sends a "turn on" signal in response to any sex-related stimulation, and sexual brakes, which send a "turn off" signal in response to any perceived threat. When people experience sexual difficulties, it's occasionally because there's not enough stimulation to the accelerator, but more often it's because there's too much stimulation to the brakes.

Some Good Questions:

- What is it that I want when I want sex?

- What is it that I like when I like sex?

- What activates my accelerator?

- What hits my brakes?

- What contexts allow for my brakes to be released?

Chapter 2

CENTER PLEASURE

When I first began having long(ish)-term sexual relationships during my college years I believed an old-fashioned narrative, which I think a lot of us are taught, about how desire works. We're told it's all passion and "spark" early in a relationship, and that lasts a couple of years maybe; then we have kids or buy a fixer-upper house or generally get busy with work and life, and the spark fizzles out, especially after fifty, when apparently every hormone we ever had floats away on a sea of aging and we're left, sexless and neutered, to hold hands at sunset. Our options, we're told, are either to accept the fizzling of our desire for sex or to fight against it, to invest our time, attention, and even our money in "keeping the spark alive."

Well, it turns out every part of that narrative is not merely wrong, but wrongheaded. A lot of books about sex in long-term relationships are about "keeping the spark alive," and they too are wrong-

headed. They're so twentieth century, with their rigid gender
scripts and cringingly oversimplified ideas about sex and evolution.

I call this mess of wrongheadedness the desire imperative.[1]

The desire imperative says:

- At the start of a sexual and/or romantic relationship,
  we should feel a "spark," a spontaneous, giddy craving
  for sexual intimacy with our (potential) partner that
  might even feel obsessive.

- The sparky desire we're supposed to feel at the beginning of a relationship is the correct, best, healthy, normal kind of desire, and if we don't have it, then we
  don't have anything worth having.

- If we have to put any preparation or planning into our
  sex lives, then we don't want it "enough."

- If our partner doesn't just spontaneously want us, out
  of the blue, without effort or preparation, on a regular
  basis, they don't want us "enough."

The desire imperative puts desire at the center of our definition
of sexual well-being. It says there is only one right way to experience desire, and without that, nothing else matters. And so people
worry about sexual desire. If desire changes or it seems to be missing, people worry that there's something very wrong. It's the most
common reason couples seek sex therapy.

Here's the irony of the desire imperative: Does all that worry
about "spark" activate the accelerator and make it easier to want
and like sex? On the contrary, worry mainly hits the brakes and
puts sex further out of reach.

But there's an alternative: Center pleasure.

Desire is not what matters. Not "passion," not "keeping the
spark alive."

Pleasure is what matters.

Center pleasure, because great sex over the long term is not about how much you want sex, it's about how much you like the sex you're having.

I'll be repeating this a lot, because we have all spent so many years soaking in the desire imperative that even people who know better (including me!) can find themselves slipping back into worry about desire.

Here's a helpful analogy about pleasure versus desire, which I learned from sex therapist Christine Hyde:

> *Imagine your best friend invites you to a party. You say yes because it's your best friend! And it's a party!*
>
> *Then as the date approaches, you start thinking,* Ugh, we have to arrange childcare . . . there's going to be so much traffic . . . am I really going to want to put on my party clothes at the end of a long week?
>
> *But you said you would go, so you arrange the childcare, you deal with the traffic, and you put on your party clothes— maybe you even bop to some fun music as you trim your ear and nose hair then don the glitter and platform heels.*
>
> *You show up to the party.*
>
> *And what happens then?*
>
> *Usually, you have fun at the party!*
>
> *If everyone's having fun at the party,* you are doing it right.

The party metaphor is a gentle, simple way to explain that sexual satisfaction is not about "spark," it's about connecting in a way that feels worthwhile to you and your partner. An even easier way to explain it is:

Pleasure is the measure.

Pleasure is the measure of sexual well-being. Like I said in the introduction, great sex over the long-term isn't about how often you do it or where you do it or with whom or in what positions or how many orgasms you have or even how enthusiastically you anticipate sex, but how much you like the sex you are having.

In this chapter, let's get clear about what we mean by "pleasure" and what we mean by "desire." After that, I'll describe why pleasure belongs at the center of our definition of sexual well-being, allowing desire to be on the periphery. By the end of this chapter, I hope you'll begin to notice when you start worrying about desire—yours or your partner's—and think instead, "Ah! There's the desire imperative again. That's my cue to center pleasure."

Spontaneous Desire vs. Responsive Desire

A simple place to start changing how we think about desire and pleasure is understanding what sex researchers and therapists say about desire. They call the "spark" of the desire imperative "spontaneous desire," and it is one of the normal ways to experience sexual desire, but it is not associated with great sex in a long-term relationship.

They also describe "responsive desire," which is not a "spark" feeling but rather an openness to exploring pleasure and seeing where it goes. It often shows up as "scheduled" sex, where you plan ahead, prepare, groom, get a babysitter, and then you show up. You put your body in the bed, you let your skin touch your partner's skin, and your body wakes up! It says, "Oh, right! I really like this! I really like this person!" *Where spontaneous desire emerges in anticipation of pleasure, responsive desire emerges in response to pleasure.*

Both are normal and neither is better than the other . . . but it's responsive desire that is associated with great sex over the long term.[2]

Responsive desire. Not "passion," not "spark," but pleasure, trust, and mutuality. That's the fundamental empirical reason to center pleasure over spark.

So, what's pleasure?

Pleasure Is *Sensation in Context*

Pleasure is the measure of sexual well-being—that is, whether or not you *like* the sex you are having. Pleasure is the measure.

So, what even is pleasure?

Well. Does a sensation feel good? How good? Does it feel bad? How bad?

That's the whole thing. Pleasure is the simplest thing in the world, in the sense of declaring whether a sensation feels good or not. Next time you're eating your very favorite food, notice what that pleasure is like—the food's appearance, its texture, aroma, and flavor. Notice what pleasure does to your body. Pleasure is simple . . .

But that doesn't mean it's always easy. We've been lied to about the nature of pleasure, just as we've been lied to about the nature of desire. We've been told that sexual pleasure is supposed to be easy and obvious, and if it's not easy and obvious, then there's something wrong. For some people, experiencing pleasure is like finding Waldo: so frustrating that you start to wonder why you're even looking.

We've been told that pleasure comes from being touched in the right place, in the right way, by the right person, and if that touch, in that place, by that person, feels good some of the time but not other times, that's a problem. These lies show up in movies and romance novels and porn, where the main characters may be running away from the villain or even just exhausted and overwhelmed by life, but Partner A touches the magic spot on Partner B's body and it doesn't matter what else is going on, Partner B's knees melt and their genitals tingle.

If that's how pleasure works for you, cool.

For the rest of us, pleasure isn't about the right place on your body touched in the right way. It's the right place, the right way, by the right person, at the right time, in the right external circumstances, and the right internal state. In short: It's *sensation in the right context.*

A simple example of this is tickling. Tickling is not everyone's favorite (though it is some people's favorite!), but you can imagine a scenario where partners are already turned on, in a trusting, playful erotic situation, and Partner A tickles Partner B and it feels good! But if those same partners are in the middle of an argument about, say, money, and Partner A tries to tickle Partner B, will that feel good? Or would Partner B feel more like punchin' somebody in the nose than snuggling?

Because pleasure is sensation in the right context, that means *any* sensation may feel good, great, spectacular, just okay, or terrible, depending on the context in which you experience it.

Conscious pleasure is different from conscious pain. Because pain is a danger signal, a warning that we may not be safe, it gets priority in our brains. Pleasure can be rewarding, but as far as our basic survival is concerned, pain takes precedence. Pain is a rude customer, pulling insistently at your attention. "Hey! Hey! Listen to me! There's a problem! Hey!" Pain is stubborn, too, often persisting long after the painful event has ended or the injury has healed. You solve the rude customer's complaint and it's not enough. Any reminder of the bad experience, and pain may start complaining all over again.

Conscious pleasure is more fragile. Pleasure is a shy animal. We can observe it from a safe distance, but if we approach too fast, it will run. If we try to capture it, it will panic. You have to build trust with your pleasure before it will allow you to observe it closely.

Pain happens when our brains interpret a signal from our bodies as a sign of danger, and our brains are more likely to interpret something as a sign of danger when there are already a lot of other signals about danger in our brains. When you're stressed, your brain is primed to interpret almost anything as a threat. When you're already in pain, other sensations are more likely to be experienced as additional pain. When you feel unsafe, sick, untrusting, threatened, or in any way at risk for harm, your brain is only too ready to interpret a sensation as uncomfortable, irritating, or even painful.

Pleasure happens when we feel safe enough. Trusting enough, healthy enough, welcome enough, at low-enough risk. Everyone's threshold for "enough" is different, and it changes from situation to situation. But when we create that safe-enough context, our brains have the capacity to interpret any sensation as pleasurable.

"Context" means both your internal state and your external circumstances. Later in this chapter, and throughout the rest of this book, we'll talk about how to create a context that grants your brain easy access to sexual pleasure. Right now, all you need to do is recognize that it is normal for a sensation to feel good today and not so good tomorrow, simply because the context changed.

Pleasure Is Not Desire
(though Desire Can Be Pleasurable)

Pleasure and desire are different systems in the brain. At the level of the emotional, mammalian brain, desire is known as "wanting" or "incentive salience," and pleasure is discussed as "liking" or hedonic impact.[3]

"Wanting," in the brain, is a vast network of dopamine-related circuitry that mediates how motivated we are to pursue a goal. "Liking," by contrast, is a set of smaller "hedonic hot spots" where opioids and endocannabinoids mediate how good a sensation feels.

Pleasure is "Oh, that's niiiiice," and "Yay!"

Desire is "Ooo*ooo*oooh, what's that?" and "How do I get more?"

Pleasure is stillness, savoring what's happening in the moment.

Desire is forward movement, exploring to create something that doesn't currently exist.

Pleasure is a perception of a sensation.

Desire is motivation toward a goal.

In a sense, pleasure is satisfaction and desire is dissatisfaction, because pleasure is enjoying an experience, while desire is motivation to pursue something different.

Here, I'll put it in a table:

PLEASURE	DESIRE
"Liking"	"Wanting"
Opiods, Endocannabinoids	Dopamine
Ahhhhh, that's nice! Yum! Yay!	Oooh, what's that? Where is it? How do I get it?
"That feels good"	"I want more"
Enjoying	Eagerness
Perception	Motivation
Hedonic impact	Incentive salience
Satisfaction	Dissatisfaction

And here's a highly simplified illustration of the neuroanatomy of "wanting" and "liking":

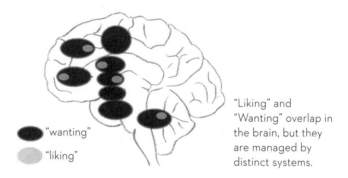

"wanting"

"liking"

"Liking" and "Wanting" overlap in the brain, but they are managed by distinct systems.

See? They're different (though overlapping) neural systems, with different (though overlapping) experiences linked to them. For sure, they are related to each other, but you can want more of something without liking it, and you can like something without wanting more of it.

Consider the "wanting" involved in continuous, joyless scrolling on social media. You're searching for something you can't name, maybe for the reward of, at last, finding something that makes you feel good or that even confirms your worst fears. You want . . . something. But you're not enjoying it, you're just following the urge to keep looking. Desire without pleasure.

Boredom, at its most uncomfortable, is wanting without liking.

Your brain is searching for something to focus on, something to do with itself. All those neurons and nothing to occupy them! It's not like daydreaming or mind-wandering, where you simply allow your brain to travel imaginary paths and feel satisfyingly occupied.

Conversely, consider the "liking" involved in being handed a gift, out of the blue. The moment of receiving the gift, even before you open it, is pleasure in the absence of desire. It is the pleasure of learning that someone was thinking of you when you weren't there.

The delight of watching your favorite people enjoying themselves together is liking without wanting. Suppose you put in the effort to throw a party, and now here they are, all your favorite people, laughing together and playing. Pleasure. Satisfaction. Because something you planned is bringing pleasure to people you love. And it doesn't even matter that that pleasure was planned rather than spontaneous.

So far, so simple.

Where it can get muddy is in how desire *feels*. Pleasure, by definition, feels good. Desire per se is more or less neutral; it's the context that makes it feel good or bad. I think people confuse desire for pleasure because desire sometimes feels good. Once we recognize that desire can also feel bad, we begin to understand both how desire and pleasure are not the same thing and why pleasure is the one that really matters.

How Sexual Desire Feels

Anticipation, expectation, craving, longing, these are all ways of experiencing desire that can feel delightful and even ecstatic. But anticipation, expectation, craving, and longing can also feel frustrating, irritating, and annoying. Desire can be hope and optimism, but it can also be anxiety and fear.

Whether desire feels good or not depends on the context. *All* pleasure depends on the context.

If you have experienced desire, stop and recall a moment when it was pleasurable. Probably, the object of your desire, whether it was a lover or a new gadget or a tasty snack, seemed within reach, maybe you felt in control of whether or not you got what you wanted, maybe your desire was grounded in a promise someone made that filled you with anticipation.

The pleasurable version of spontaneous desire is, I think, why people get confused about the difference between pleasure and desire and why we might be convinced that "spontaneous" is the good, right, normal kind of desire. After all, it was "easy"—or at least, it happened out of nowhere—and it was fun.

But spontaneous sexual desire can feel terrible, too. Suppose you can't figure out how to get closer to your object of desire, or the object of your desire is entirely out of reach or, worse, actively rejecting you, pushing you away. In that context, your ongoing desire can feel like a form of torture.

If you've wanted to want sex, you've experienced a different uncomfortable desire. Many people who struggle to let go of the "ideal" of spontaneous desire know how awful it feels to want something you can't get, which is why it's so important that we remind ourselves that it's responsive desire, not spontaneous desire, that characterizes great sex over the long term. If you enjoy the sex you have, you're already doing it right, and you're allowed to stop trying to create spontaneous desire.

If we think only about the pleasurable experiences of desire, we end up using the words "pleasure" and "desire" more or less interchangeably. But they're different; we know they're different because of the brain science. And if pleasure always is pleasurable but desire is only sometimes pleasurable, doesn't it make sense to center pleasure, and allow desire to emerge in contexts that maximize the chances that the desire will feel good?

Are You Still Worried about Spontaneous Desire?

If I wanted to spark controversy, I'd say there's no such thing as a sexual desire problem, and all the news articles and think pieces and self-help books and medical research focused on a "cure" for low desire are irrelevant. The "cure" for low desire is pleasure. When we put pleasure at the center of our definition of sexual well-being, we eliminate any need to worry about desire.

But I'm not here for controversy, I'm here to make your sex life better. So I'll just say: Don't sweat desire. If you're worried about your partner's low desire, ask them about pleasure. If you're worried about your own low desire, talk to your partner about pleasure. You'll find lots of tools for these conversations throughout the book. Desire can be a fun bonus extra; it's as important as simultaneous orgasms, which is to say, a neat party trick but *not remotely necessary* for a satisfying long-term sex life.

And yet. In my unscientific survey of a few hundred strangers, some people reported that what they want when they want sex is spontaneity:

> *"I hate talking about having sex before I have sex. Like if it can't happen naturally, I kinda don't want it."*

Oof, that word. "Naturally."

If the idea of talking about sex, or making a plan before you have it, feels "unnatural," hi, hello! Welcome! This section of the book is here to acknowledge the reality that talking about sex might deflate spontaneous desire, but also to ask you to consider the possibility that planning sex can be part of the pleasure and talking about sex is not just natural, it's part of the erotic connection between you and a partner.

Maybe every sexual experience you've had in response to spontaneous desire has been better than any sex you've ever had in response to a plan. But did you really not plan before any of that great "spontaneous" sex? When you're in a new or emerging relationship, do you not spend time daydreaming about a hot date, making plans for dinner or an adventure together, exchanging flirtatious texts, emails, phone calls, whispers? Hot-and-heavy, falling-in-love horniness is often accompanied by a *lot* of planning and preparation and, yes, even talking about sex in advance. Do you not spend time getting ready for it, grooming, dressing carefully, making sure you smell good?

Is that . . . "natural"?

The myth that the "natural" way to have sex is for it to be spontaneously borne of mutual horniness, without having to talk about it or make a plan? That's the desire imperative I described at the start of this chapter. The desire imperative insists that without spontaneous desire, we don't want sex "enough." If we have to plan it, there's a problem.

But consider what our lives are like—what our contexts are like. We schedule large portions of our days, often weeks or even months in advance. We fill our calendars with work and school and family and friends and entertainment. We fill our bodies with stress and a sense of obligation to others and to ourselves. We impose modern exigencies that don't even create adequate opportunity for natural sleep, much less unplanned yet mutually enthusiastic sex.

I'd like people who adore spontaneity to consider the possibility that spontaneity matters less than pleasure. To that end, I want to acknowledge the real phenomenon of spontaneous desire potentially evaporating when you talk about sex. It's true. I've felt it . . . and I want to show you how little it matters.

Back in my twenties, I had an on-again, off-again relationship with someone I'll call Coen (not his real name). At a certain point, we agreed we would stop having sex because it was only making our lives more complicated and miserable. Then, inevitably, one night after a party, I went back to his place for coffee and a chat, and he made a move.

Honestly, it was sexy. I felt all the excitement of "I want to, but I shouldn't."

But we'd had good reasons for our decision to stop having sex. My "I shouldn't" wasn't just a playful "Ooh, I'm a bad girl," it was a "We are going to damage each other badly if we do this"; a "We are going to break each other's hearts. Again."

So instead of kissing him back, I said, "We decided not to do this."

And Coen said, "But what if just this once?"

While he kissed my neck, I reiterated the reasons we had decided not to do this. For example, he was still in love with his ex.

As he had said himself, over and over, when he had sex with some-one he habitually fell into the role of boyfriend, so I'd feel like he was acting like my boyfriend and he'd feel like he was waiting for his ex to come back. So not only were we totally unable to meet each other's needs as romantic partners, we were destroying the friendship we had had before we started having sex.

Coen said, "What if we agree that I won't do that?"

Valiantly resisting the pull of desire, I said, "Can you? Because I am too busy and too exhausted to go through that again."

He actually thought about it. And he said, "Yes."

And I believed him.

Now, in a romance novel or a TV show what would happen next is we'd both feel set free from the ambivalence that was holding us back and we'd slam our bodies together like we'd each been re-leased from a slingshot. In a way, I wish that were what had hap-pened, because then I could say, "See? Talking about it makes it *extra horny*!"

But in real life, the opposite happened.

My ambivalence had been hot air keeping the balloon of my lust swollen and ready. When I resolved my ambivalence by talking about it, my horniness deflated. Coen stood up to go lock his apart-ment door, and by the time he got back, seconds later, I felt neutral about having sex.

What would you think, in a moment like that? Would you worry that something had gone wrong? Would you decide the sex wasn't worth having if the pulsing horniness evaporated? Would you wish you hadn't protected you and your partner from un-wanted consequences if it meant preserving the spontaneity? I'm sure the person who wrote, "If it can't happen naturally, I kinda don't want it," would have stopped everything there. No sex for them that night.

But my story doesn't end with the deflating of my spontaneous desire. Coen and I did have sex that night, and it was really fun; it was playful instead of desperate. Rather than just getting naked right there in the living room, as we would have had to do in order to avoid confronting the real choice we were making, I asked him to drag me into his bedroom by one ankle. And the next day, he did not fall into his old habits.

It worked out this way because I had already begun deconstructing the desire imperative in my own life. It's true that talking about it and resolving the "we want to but we shouldn't" ambivalence drained away my hot craving, but even then I knew *that's not a bad thing.*

So even though I can't say, "See? Talking about it makes it extra horny!" I can say, "See? Talking about it makes it more fun *and* you don't have to worry about the consequences later." When you center pleasure, instead of desire, you have access to pleasurable experiences that minimize the risk of unwanted consequences.

Imagine if it hadn't been emotional consequences but physical health or social consequences that I was considering. Suppose I had said, "This is very hot, but do you have a condom?"

Or ". . . but I need to pause and get some lube."

Or ". . . isn't your other relationship monogamous?"

Or even just "Hey, can you check that the door is locked?"

Any of these can deflate spontaneity. But imagine the unwanted consequences people experience if they follow the desire imperative. Sexually transmitted infection, unwanted pregnancy, damage to your reputation, hurting someone's feelings, having your own feelings hurt, these and more are all real and important potential consequences that deserve priority over protecting "spontaneity."

A lot of sex educators say that "interrupting" sex this way, to talk about something like birth control or STI prevention or other emotional or physical safety issues, doesn't impact desire, and I'm sure for some people it doesn't. But for other people, people like me, it may impact desire. But that's no big deal, because desire is not the point. *Pleasure* is the point.

I don't expect you to believe me right away. I know you've been taught to worry about desire. It might even feel troubling or problematic to say that desire doesn't matter. Maybe you're thinking, *What could you possibly mean, Emily, to not worry about not wanting it and just enjoy it instead? Are you telling me to enjoy sex I don't want???*

On the contrary! I'm saying: Imagine a world where all of us *only ever have sex we enjoy*. And anything we don't enjoy, we just don't do! We don't do it, *and*—get this—we don't worry about not doing it! When we put pleasure at the center of our definition of sexual well-being, sex we don't like is never even on the table.

Mike and Kendra

I didn't know Mike and Kendra at the beginning of their struggles, I only met them at the end. It took them some time and several different approaches before they found all the tools they needed, but I guarantee you they found their happily ever after.

The nature of their struggle? Mike wanted Kendra to want him, spontaneously and passionately. She used to. Early in their relationship, she experienced spontaneous desire often and easily. But for the last four years, she almost never felt spontaneous desire. That change began with her first, quite difficult pregnancy and continued through the second, easier pregnancy, breastfeeding, and weening of their second child, now a one-year-old toddler.

For four years, they had been having sex when he wanted it or when she felt so guilty that she initiated. This isn't even close to a worst-case scenario for a couple like this, but when I finally heard what they had been going through, I felt heartbroken for them.

Mike wanted to feel wanted again.

On one level, of course he did! It's one of The Big Four, the most common things people want when they want sex with a partner. Heck, who doesn't want to be wanted? And Kendra had wanted him, spontaneously and passionately, at the beginning of their relationship.

But on another level, they liked the sex they had, when they had it, and, as Kendra pointed out sometimes, if he didn't make such a big deal about spontaneous desire, they would literally not have a problem.

They are not people who fight. Yelling is not their style.

They prefer to sit down and have conversations and listen to each other's feelings and try to find common ground. They read Come as You Are, *and Kendra really wanted to incorporate the idea of responsive desire into their approach to sex, but Mike was mostly interested in ways to create spontaneous desire for Kendra. They discussed this difference calmly and reasonably . . . over and over . . . for years.*

Can you feel how focused all of that is on desire? On "fixing" Kendra so that she has the desire experience Mike wants her to have?

At the start of their journey, Kendra tried a thought experiment. One night when they were lying in bed together, having not had sex again, she said, "Can it be enough sometimes if we just enjoy it, without having to be super horny for each other? Can it be enough that I really like sex with you, even when I'm not turned on before we start?"

"But how can we really like the sex if we don't want it first?"

"Dude," Kendra said, "I do it all the time."

"What?"

"All the time! If I'm just in a good mood and I know it'll make you happy if I initiate, I go ahead and flirt with you and kiss you and enjoy it, and we have sex and it feels great and I'm like, 'Wow, I'm glad we did that. We should do that again sometime.'"

Mike nodded and thought. Then he said, "That doesn't seem right, that we just have a nice time together. We should be hot for each other, like we can't wait. Like it was before."

"Sure, a longer-term goal, but I want to think about what would happen if, for the time being, we just really enjoy each other, without needing to change anything? What if, in this season of our life, enjoying each other is enough?"

Silence from Mike as he processed.

Kendra added, "Because spontaneous desire is not some-

thing I seem to have any control over, but pleasure is. And imagine if I was like, 'I only want to have sex when you don't have spontaneous desire. Stop experiencing spontaneous desire so we can have truly great sex.' Wouldn't that feel terrible?"

"But that's just never a problem. How does my desire have anything to do with yours?"

This was the point when Kendra's emotional energy ran out. She said, "Well, maybe your constant spontaneous desire is creating a lot of pressure for me and actually makes it more difficult for me to experience it myself."

"But that's crazy. This is just how I am, and you used to be like this, too. Something happened. Something went wrong."

Kendra sighed and said, "Okay. Well, maybe think about it."

Let's just notice what a heroic effort she put into being extremely calm. This is the emotional labor that so many women put into their relationships, especially those with men.[4]

She could have said, "No, you're crazy. It's crazy to think that just because I changed there's something wrong. Everything in our lives changed, and I changed with it. Maybe there's something wrong with you, that you're not adapting at all." But obviously it's just as not-okay for her to call him crazy as it was for him to call her crazy.

She could have said, "How does your desire have anything to do with mine? Are you kidding? How does my desire have anything to do with yours, you stinkin' hypocrite?" But she knew that kind of criticism and contempt would have raised his defenses, which wouldn't help them make progress.

She didn't say these things, because they're not people who "fight."

But also, Mike could have said, "Huh. I'm starting to notice that my investment in your spontaneous desire isn't really about what I want for you, it's about what I want for me. If I can focus instead on your pleasure, for you, that would take away the pressure that might actually be making it more difficult for me to have what I want."

He could have said, "Well, we've been trying it my way without success for a long time now. How about we try it your way and see what happens? I feel like the worst thing that can happen is we have some sex we enjoy, and the best thing that could happen is we have sex we enjoy so much that you start wanting it more often!"

But he didn't, because neither of them yet saw the towering external force that was obstructing their view of the solution to their struggles.

It would take many more conversations before they made the shift to centering pleasure and co-creating a pleasure-positive context. Both of them had spent their entire adult lives believing that "spark" and "passion" are the defining characteristics of a great sex life. It takes time to shift to a fundamentally different way of understanding sexuality.

Context Is a "Third Thing"

The rest of this book is about co-creating, with a long-term partner, a context that makes pleasure easier.

And yes indeed, I'm going to be suggesting that you talk with your partner about context. I'm going to suggest so much talking, that, if I do my job right, you may spend more time talking with your partner about sex than you spend doing it. It's not always easy to talk about sex, and I'll offer tools to make it easier in part 2 of the book. But getting to know each other's contexts is an essential part of building a satisfying sexual connection that can last decades. It will take more talking early in the process, as you explore and learn about your own, your partner's, and your shared contexts. Gradually, you'll come to know each other so well, much can go unspoken.

I think people's difficulty talking about sex is related to how they feel about pleasure and desire. If you buy into the desire imperative, you may have become convinced that if you have to talk about it, there must be a problem. And that's just not true; couples with great long-term sexual connections talk about sex.[5] Or if you've been taught to feel shame around pleasure, then talking about what you want and like may feel inherently shameful, even with the person with whom you share those pleasures. Releasing yourself from the desire imperative and from pleasure shame are not changes that will happen today. They will happen little by little, as you step outside your cultural learning, into the sunlight of your shared pleasures.

To make it a little easier, I suggest you try to replace the idea of sexual desire with the idea of sexual *interest*. To me, sexual interest is sexual *curiosity*. You're probably reading this book because you are interested in sex, even if you don't currently desire it. You are curious. You want to learn more, dive deeper, discover ways to create positive change or to cope with unwanted change. Hi, hello! Is your partner also interested in sex—by which I mean, do they find sex interesting? Remember, the couples who sustain a strong sexual connection over multiple decades are not the ones who crave the sex, they're friends who decide that sex matters in their relationship. They're interested in sex, curious about it. It's important to them, in all its expansive variety.

I've started thinking of the shared project of creating a great context for sex as a "third thing," something both partners are interested in and want to spend time on. I get this term from poet Donald Hall, who wrote of his twenty-three-year marriage to poet Jane Kenyon in an essay titled "The Third Thing":

> *We did not spend our days gazing into each other's eyes. We did that gazing when we made love or when one of us was in trouble, but most of the time our gazes met and entwined as they looked at a third thing. Third things are essential to marriages, objects or practices or habits or arts or institutions or games or human beings that provide a site of joint rapture or contentment.*[6]

A third thing is a shared interest, like your favorite TV show or your love of sushi or the sports team to which you're loyal or the parties you throw together. What do you and your long-term partner do with the time you have chosen to spend together? What are your third things, your "sites of joint rapture or contentment"? It could be your kids or the works of Frida Kahlo or women's soccer or the vegetable patch in your yard or swing dancing or LARPing or your special-needs cat. And it could be the co-creation of contexts that make it easier to experience pleasure.

I believe your shared context is worthy of your shared attention, a third thing that holds your mutual interest. Paying ongoing attention to context allows you to assess and adjust your lives and your relationship.

This is not sexual desire itself, in the way we're used to thinking about desire. It's being interested in sex and in each other. It's being interested in pleasure.

Maybe think about it this way:

Spontaneous desire is like knowing there's cake in the fridge, a delicious, gorgeous cake, your desire for which has nothing to do with hunger and everything to do with the delight of that mouthful of glorious flavor. Maybe you wake up in the middle of the night and your first thought is *There's cake in the fridge!* There's nothing wrong with spontaneous desire; cake is delicious. (Though if you're gluten-sensitive, your longing for the cake is a torment, not a delight. Context changes everything.)

Responsive desire is like showing up to a party where there's delicious, delicious cake—sure, it might start out feeling like you're just showing up because you said you would, but once you're there and you hear the beat of the music and you see the laughing faces of your favorite people, you join in with pleasure.

Then there are the couples who center pleasure by co-creating a context that makes pleasure easy. In terms of the party metaphor, they don't just show up, they *love to entertain.*[7] When they're at the grocery store, they consider what's necessary to keep their fridge stocked with everything they need to create a beautiful charcuterie board, bruschetta, fresh guacamole. As they get ready for the party, they take time to lay the mortadella in beautiful little heaps on a handmade board they bought with their partner at the farmer's market they explored on a vacation fifteen years ago. They mound the goat cheese in a pretty depression glass sherbet bowl, inherited from a beloved friend. They place a long sprig of rosemary across the basket of freshly baked rolls, still steaming from the oven.

Why take time to make a meal beautiful? Why think ahead as you write a grocery list for a get-together you don't even know for sure you'll have? Maybe some people put in that kind of effort simply to show off or impress people. But for people who prioritize sharing pleasure with loved ones, all that effort is part of the pleasure you anticipate sharing. You put in the extra forethought because that's how much you care about creating pleasure to share.

In concrete terms, responsive desire might look like this: You show up to a scheduled date night, stressed and distracted but glad to be there. You let your skin touch your partner's skin, and your body wakes up and goes, "Oh right! I like this! I like this person! What a good idea this is!"

But when you center pleasure, you plan ahead, adjusting your schedule so that you have a minimum of stress on the day of the date and considering what your partner might need in order to be in a great state of mind on that day. Centering pleasure is finishing the laundry and the dishes, to minimize distractions, and cleaning the bathtub so your partner can have a relaxing bath. Above all, centering pleasure looks like asking your partner what helps them to feel cared for, attended to, and wanted; it looks like sharing with your partner what helps you to feel cared for, attended to, and wanted.

You are probably not aroused as you do those dishes. You probably don't feel horny as you scrub the ring of soap scum from the tub. You are not "in the mood." But you don't have to be in the mood for your best friend's birthday party while you plan it, you don't have to feel like going to your kid's martial arts competition to order an ice cream cake for the day. You don't need a mood. You need to care. It needs to matter to you.

We plan and prepare for so many things that matter in our lives.

Why would we believe that sex should just happen, without effort? And why, if sex matters to us and our relationships, would we not want to put whatever effort we can into making it a delight?

Not all the sex in your relationship needs to be an event, of course. When I say "center pleasure" or "co-create a context that makes it easier to access pleasure," sometimes that means planning an event, but sometimes it means out-of-the-blue little erotic encounters that "just happen," because you've put time and effort into creating a context that makes it easy for them to happen.

Assess the Context

If pleasure is the shy animal I described before, appearing only in the right context and staying only when we approach gently and observe it calmly, what is the "right" context?

The rest of this book is all about understanding what contexts make it easy for your brain to access pleasure, what context you're currently in, and how to create change in your context.

Here, let's begin with a simple exercise. First, think of a specific experience when you had easy, abundant pleasure, and consider what aspects of the context made accessing pleasure easy. Don't fall into the desire imperative's trap of imagining an experience when you had a lot of spontaneous desire—your easy pleasure may coincidentally have been accompanied by desire, but it's not the desire that matters.

If you've never experienced easy, abundant pleasure, you can imagine a situation that you expect might make pleasure easy.

Context is made of a combination of internal state and external circumstances. The next chapter, "Your Emotional Floorplan," is all about your internal state, so for now let's consider external circumstances. This includes things like your relationship with your partner, the setting, and other life factors like stress about your job or worry about money, your family, and the state of the world.

Relationship issues were the contextual factor that I fixed with Coen, that moment many years ago, when my desire faded but my pleasure expanded. In your experience of easy pleasure, how was your relationship with the partner with whom you shared that pleasure?

External factors also include the *setting* where sex happens. Setting is what mattered for the couple who built their bed into the wall. Are you at home, in your shared bed with your certain special someone? Are you on vacation together? Are you in front of your screen at one end of a wireless internet connection, while your partner is at the other end? Are you in the bathroom at your favorite nightclub? The settings that make it easier for your brain to access pleasure will vary from person to person and relationship to relationship. And it's important to note that a fantasy context may be entirely different from a real-life context. If the fantasy of the bathroom at your favorite nightclub opens up your brain's access to pleasure, that doesn't mean that the reality of that bathroom will have the same effect.

Even small adjustments to a real setting can make a difference. For example, when I was struggling, my spouse and I realized we could remove one barrier to sex by making it easier to close the bedroom door. Most of the time, we kept the door propped open with a small linen chest, so the dogs could come and go, but during sexy times we opted to keep the dogs out of the room. Closing the door required moving the chest and then pulling up a large corner of rug to get it out of the path of the door. It was a minor hassle with a simple solution: We removed the rug and the little chest, propping the door with a small, easy to move wastebasket instead.

Also: sex towels. Our sex sometimes involves some bodily fluids, and *wiping* is often part of afterplay. It's not super-sexy to have to get out of bed, dripping with fluids, and go into the bathroom to get a towel, especially on a cold New England night. Solution: We allocated a drawer, reachable from the bed, to fill with towels dedicated to sex. Some problems are just that easy to solve. Move a piece of furniture. Put some linens in a different drawer. These were small changes to our setting that made a noticeable difference.

When you've got a sense of the context that made it easy for your brain to access pleasure, try thinking about your current context. How's your relationship? What's your setting? How are you feeling about the state of the world?

And . . . how do you feel about pleasure? Pleasure feels good, but how do you feel about feeling good?

How Do You Feel about Pleasure?

This is a too-often ignored factor that I want to emphasize early. *How do you feel* about pleasure itself, especially sexual pleasure?

Just as we were lied to about pleasure, told that it was obvious and easy, we were lied to about *how to feel* about pleasure. Too many of us were taught to fear, resent, or otherwise disparage pleasure.

The late, great sex educator Betty Dodson encountered this often, as she coached many women to orgasm. Her "rock 'n' roll" method taught women to ride the visceral wave of arousal and orgasm, as pleasure rolled through them like a rising tide. She made a series of instructional videos showing women's evolving relationships with their own sexual pleasure.

In one video, one of Betty's clients, Cynthia, age forty-one, isn't sure if she was having orgasms or, if she *was* having them, thought they were small, almost-nothing orgasms.

"What I picture it being like or I think it should be like, is just bigger, all over bigger and more where you're just out of control and you're . . . just . . . very dramatic."

Betty assures her, "You're never out of control. [. . .] You're in your body; the only thing you're out of is you're out of your mind."

Early in her coached masturbation session, Cynthia tells Betty that the lowest setting of the vibrator is good and she doesn't want lube. Eventually, though, Betty directly invites more intense vibration and lube.

Immediately, Cynthia recognizes, "That's better."

"Hang on it, oh, hang on it," Betty coaches her, as Cynthia's moans crescendo.

After Cynthia's second orgasm, she describes her revelation: "I never let [the vibrator] stay on long enough. . . . Instead of backing off when it feels so intense, I just kept it there and that's when it gets very . . . When you *meet it,* it feels like it really changes the whole thing. . . . It felt like, 'Oh, I have to take it away, it's too much,' but it isn't too much."

"That's the most important thing to learn," Betty praises. "When it gets really strong, move into it.

"Meet it," Betty tells her. "Get in it."

Throughout her session, Cynthia has, by my count, at least three orgasms. The barrier to her pleasure was her uncertainty in the face of pleasure that felt so good it seemed like "too much."

This is the story of our relationships with pleasure. We feel like it's too much; it's not too much. When pleasure feels strong, you don't have to move away from it.

Over and over in Betty's sessions, women learn that the urge to take away stimulation when it feels like "too much" can interrupt pleasure and prevent it from growing into all that it can be in their bodies. "Stay on it. Don't stop. Keep it there," Betty tells her clients and us. "Meet the intensity with your intensity. Move into it instead of pulling away from it. Ride it. Hang on to it."

In another memorable scene, Lisa, a client who is exploring her way toward her first orgasm from masturbation, gets to an intense level of arousal, at the pulsing edge of orgasm, and her response is to pull the vibrator away from her clitoris.

"Don't stop," says Betty, guiding the vibrator back to her client's mons.

"Sorry," Lisa says, and she holds the vibrator against her body again. Because of course she apologizes.

"Stay on it," Betty coaches. "Stay on it."

Seconds later, we see the unmistakable body-shaking pulses of tension taking Lisa's body like a riptide. With Betty's encouragement, Lisa moans and then screams her pleasure, allowing it to be as big as it wants, to last as long as it wants.

In this video, we witness the moment when Lisa learns how to be still with pleasure, not to run from it and not to try for it, but to *allow* it. To meet it.

How do you feel about your own pleasure? When you're experiencing intense sexual sensations in a safe-enough context, do you sometimes turn away from it, to diminish it? Let me name the emotion: To worry that a sexual sensation might overwhelm you or be "too much" is to *fear* pleasure.

Pleasure is not unsafe. You can allow your body to experience all the pleasure you choose to create. As Lama Rod Owens writes in *Love and Rage,* "Loving pleasure means that I allow it to be itself. I enjoy it when it arises and I let it go when it leaves."

The most common reason a couple seeks sex therapy is because of problems with sexual desire. So let's imagine a couple who comes to therapy with Peggy Kleinplatz, therapist, sex researcher, and co-author of *Magnificent Sex.*

One partner in this therapy session says, "I would be fine if we never had sex again. I'm sorry it makes my partner feel bad, but I just have no interest."

Her response: "Tell me more about this sex you don't want."

Inevitably, the sex they describe is "dismal and disappointing." Sex by rote. Sex where the partner doesn't feel attended to. Sex where they don't feel trusting and connected, but rather like they're exposing the bare minimum of their most authentic selves—or worse, they feel they have to pretend to be someone they are not. Sex that feels like one partner is a sex vending machine.

Peggy replies, "Well, I rather enjoy sex, but if I was having the sex you described, I wouldn't want it either."

Let's pause for a moment to appreciate the jaw-dropping simplicity of this idea:

It is *normal* not to want sex you do not like.

If the sex available to you is painful, boring, lonely, or a show you put on for someone else's pleasure, then of course you don't want it. You are not broken. Your sexual desire is not broken. It is normal to not want sex you do not enjoy, and it is normal to not want sex in a context that creates no space for your erotic self.

Then Peggy asks the gut-punch question: "What kind of sex is *worth wanting?*"

The answer, broadly speaking, is sex you *enjoy.* Sex that brings you pleasure.

So when people struggle with sexual desire, the question to ask is not "Why don't I want sex?" it's "*How do I create pleasure?*"

But there are other couples who know they'd like it if they could bring themselves to do it, but they just . . . can't. They're stuck. That was me and my spouse. I was stuck.

Stuck where, though? What does that mean? And how do you get unstuck?

That's what the next two chapters will tell us.

Chapter 2 tl;dr:

- Pleasure is the measure of sexual well-being—not how much you crave it, not how often you do it or with whom or where, or how many orgasms you have. It's whether or not you like the sex you're having. Pleasure is sensation in context; context is a combination of external circumstances and internal state.

- The "desire imperative" is a cultural narrative that says our experience of spontaneous desire is the single most important measure of our sexual functioning.

- Spontaneous desire is normal; it emerges in anticipation of pleasure. Responsive desire is also normal; it emerges in response to pleasure.

- For many "low desire" couples, the difficulty is not so much that they don't *want* the sex available to them;

it's that they don't like it—if they don't like it, of course they don't want it. Again, pleasure is the measure.

• Partners in a sexual connection can treat context as a "third thing," a site of mutual curiosity and exploration. Couples who sustain a strong sexual connection co-create a context that makes pleasure easier to access.

Some Good Questions:

• In what contexts can my brain most easily experience pleasure?

• What kind of sexual experiences have I enjoyed in the past?

• What does the pleasurable experience of sexual desire feel like for me? In what contexts do I experience it?

• In what contexts do I feel the uncomfortable experience of sexual desire (or desire for desire)?

• How do we as a couple create a context that makes it easy to access pleasure?

Chapter 3

YOUR EMOTIONAL FLOORPLAN

When I was struggling in my own long-term sexual connection, I felt *stuck*.

In terms of the party metaphor, my partner and I both knew that if we could get to the party, we would have fun . . . but it just felt like *so much effort* to get off the sofa and into bed.

"I love you," my metaphorical self would say to my party-throwing partner, "and I love going to parties with you. I just . . ." (I flop onto the sofa, magically transitioning into my comfiest pajamas on the way down, like a TikTok video) ". . . I can't."

I was stuck on this metaphorical sofa, stuck in my pajamas, stuck in a state of mind that made sexual pleasure feel a million miles away.

My stuckness was difficult for my partner, too. Everyone has a bad day or week or month, but when it happens over and over again, you, the party-throwing friend, might start to have some feelings about how your friend just . . . can't. You might start to feel like your friend doesn't care enough to try. You might feel like, well, if your friend can't be bothered to show up then maybe you shouldn't invite this friend to parties anymore. You might begin to worry that your friend doesn't enjoy the parties, or that your friend doesn't love you enough to show up to the party, that there's something wrong with the relationship itself.

Of course, I wasn't literally stuck on the sofa, I was stuck somewhere in my emotional brain and I couldn't find my way out of it and into an erotic space in my mind.

Maybe you're in a similar boat. Maybe you like the sex you would be having if only you could bring yourself to have it, but you're swamped with overwhelm, exhaustion, stress, depression, anxiety, repressed rage (we've all got it).

Or maybe you're stuck in a role that's incompatible with erotic connection—you're always in parent mode or caretaking mode or job mode. If that's the case, your problem is not your lack of desire, it's your *stuckness*. If you're stuck, no wonder you can't want sex.

To get unstuck, I learned to map my "emotional floorplan," understanding how I might get from wherever I was—physically exhausted, anxious, frustrated—to a sexy state of mind.

And that's what I want you to do.

In this chapter, you'll develop a kind of map of the different emotional states that exist in your brain, that will show you how to navigate those spaces to find yourself in the vicinity of the erotic. These rooms include seven "core" or "primary" emotional spaces in your brain.

Four of the seven systems are what I'll call "pleasure-favorable," meaning they are spaces where it's easier to access pleasure. They generally feel good and we are motivated to experience them—LUST, PLAY, SEEKING, and CARE. And three systems are "pleasure-adverse," meaning they are spaces where pleasure seems far away. They generally feel uncomfortable and we are motivated to avoid them—PANIC/GRIEF, FEAR, and RAGE.[1] Jaak Panksepp, the father of affective neuroscience and the researcher who developed this framework, put the terms in ALL CAPS to differentiate them from the day-to-day meanings of these words.[2] It's not "lust," in the ordinary sense of a person's experience of sexual desire, but rather LUST, in the technical sense of the network of brain systems whose activation generates mammalian behaviors and experiences related to courtship and sexual behavior.

To these seven emotional spaces, I will add two "bonus" spaces—the THINKING MIND, or the OFFICE, where you plan and reason, and OBSERVATIONAL DISTANCE or the scenic viewpoint, for noticing your own internal experience with nonjudgment. The seven primary emotional spaces, plus the bonus spaces, comprise much of our *internal context.*

We're going to think of these spaces as the "rooms" in your brain, laid out in an emotional floorplan. At any given moment, you are in one room or between rooms. And depending on where you are in your emotional floorplan, making your way to the vicinity of the LUST room can be easy or difficult.

In this floorplan, CARE and PLAY are the spaces that open into LUST. Sometimes it's easy to get from CARE to LUST (when you're already up in the loft), and sometimes it takes a little intentional effort to get there (when you're on the ground floor and have to climb the stairs into the loft).

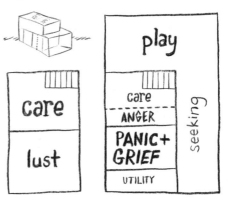

Some readers will use the floorplan pretty literally, creating an architectural map of the spaces and how they relate to each of the other spaces. I've included several illustrations as examples throughout this chapter. But some readers, maybe those who think more verbally or emotionally than spatially, may prefer to think of the floorplan as a dreamspace, where they transition from one space to another without logic or order, where different emotional spaces appear around them spontaneously and shift in ways a room in the waking world never could.

Some readers may find the floorplan metaphor doesn't work for them; you'll find some alternatives in this endnote.[3] The floorplan isn't what matters—it's just a metaphor for the actual hardware of your emotional brain. If you can identify the emotions in yourself and understand what moves you into and out of these states, that's what matters. A few of us nerdy authors, like John Gottman and Nan Wise, have been gently pushing Panksepp's model into the mainstream, because we believe it can help people in their daily lives.[4] In understanding that these different systems co-exist in our brains, we can notice how we and our loved ones move from one mental state to another. Then, whenever we're interested in transitioning from one space to another, or our partner asks us for help in transitioning, we know how. The goal, regardless of your preferred metaphor, is to trace the ways you transition into an erotic state of mind, from some other state of mind. Pay attention to which transitions are most effortless and which most effortful.

Fair warning: This is the longest and most sciencey chapter. But it changes people's lives, it changes how people understand themselves and their partners as erotic beings. I have done my best to make it accessible and easy to apply to your life.

It's a lot, but it's worth it.

Let's go room by room in your mental floorplan and find out what each space is like and how they all relate to one another.

The Pleasure-Favorable Spaces

LUST

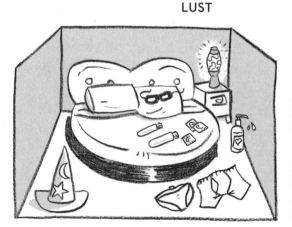

LUST is the space of courtship and sexuality. In humans, it's a highly social space and is most often surrounded by the other pleasure-favorable, highly social spaces of CARE and PLAY.

LUST is everything from sexual attraction through arousal, desire, and orgasm. It's a mental space in which any and every sensation may be interpreted as erotic.

What are some things that activate LUST inside you? What causes sexual pleasure to rise? When is it easy to allow desire to grow?

Though LUST's evolutionary origin is reproduction, humans, along with a variety of other mammals, go to the LUST space for lots of reasons, most of them nonreproductive, many of them *social*. For most people, the LUST space in our emotional brains is adjacent to the other three pleasure-favorable emotional spaces, SEEKING, PLAY, and CARE—all of which I'll discuss in more detail in the sections that follow. Most often, the way we get to a LUSTful state of mind is by going through one of these three spaces.

Can you think of a time when the transition to sexual desire was easy—when initiation happened without anyone having to worry or try hard? When pleasure happened without effort? What was happening in the minutes, hours, and even days leading up to the shift into the erotic?

How do you feel about your LUST space? While we've been taught to have feelings about many of the spaces in our emotional floorplan, LUST may be the one we've most likely been taught to feel ashamed of, not least because we were taught to be ashamed of pleasure.[5]

For people with consistently lower sexual desire than their partner, you may feel like a failure or a bad person, because you can't find your way into LUST. For those with consistently higher desire, you may feel like a bad person because LUST seems ever present. The most important thing to remember is that there is no "correct" level of desire and you have nothing to feel ashamed of about your LUST space.

The highest-desire person I've ever talked to could have sex and, mere minutes later, be just as interested in having sex as she was before she and her partner started. Nothing—not stress, not pregnancy, not illness, nothing—made her desire for sex go away. Over time, and with the help of a loving partner, she has learned she need not feel ashamed of her desire. She told me:

"I have felt shame around how important sex is to me, without a doubt. Every partner I've ever been with has had a lower sex drive. But I know I'd rather have really good, into-it sex once a week, once a month, than sex where my partner's totally checked out twice a week. I've come to a place where I actively work to make sure my partner doesn't feel obligated to have sex with me. We get there through a lot of talking, which I'm not a fan of, but we have those conversations where I'm able to iterate and reiterate, if you don't want to have sex with me, I'd rather not have sex with you."

She learned that she was not entitled to sex just because she wanted it, and that sex with partners who were there out of a sense of obligation was not sex worth having. In her relationship now, she and her wife have a clear understanding: There is no obligation, ever, there's just an open door and a welcome mat, always.

As you consider the LUST space in your emotional mind, ask yourself the questions:

- How do you know you're in that space?

- What happens in your body, thoughts, and emotions when you're there?

- How do you feel about this space?

- What pulls you into that space, and what pushes you out?

PLAY

In our daily lives, we might describe the PLAY space in our minds with words like "fun" or "joy." But more technically, PLAY is *activity done with no immediate purpose, for its own sake, just because everyone involved likes it.* You can recognize PLAY by the facial and vocal reactions of participants—laughter, smiles, wide open mouths, cheering. When you're in PLAY, there is nothing at stake, only fun to be had.

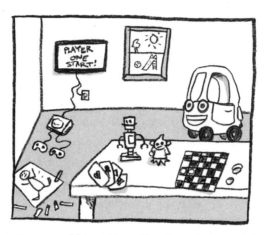

PLAY is the space of friendship and laughter, singing and dancing,
games of all kinds, with zero stakes.

PLAY can be a lot of things. There is rough-and-tumble play, like
dogs or children chasing each other and wrestling. There's fantasy
play, like children playing dress-up and inventing stories. There's
word play, like jokes, rhymes, and rhythms. Freestyle rap battles are
play. Singing, dancing, and chanting are play. The internet meme
that "queefing" (vaginal farts) is "when the small unicorn that lives
inside your vagina sneezes," that's play, too, taking something people sometimes feel embarrassed or even ashamed about, and turning it into a giggle.

There's object and sensory play—everything from splashing in
the bath or a pool to doing jigsaw puzzles. Once we know what an
object is (through SEEKING exploration), we transition to "What
can I make this object do?" or "What can I do with this object?" We
manipulate our environment with our bodies to see what happens,
and when something unexpected but safe happens, we feel the
thrill of discovery. In all its various forms, PLAY is the foundation of
friendship.

If you have gotten to LUST through PLAY, maybe you and your
partner were playing literal games, whether physical sports or
Bananagrams. Maybe you were roughhousing, and the physical
touch and heavy breathing changed the mood. The laughter and

friendship-building of PLAY might be the most underrated yet common paths to LUST.

Manual and oral sex, at their best, can be object play, activity done with no immediate purpose, for its own sake, just because everyone involved likes it, in which we explore our partner's genitals to see what happens when we try certain movements at different speeds or with different pressure. "What can I make this object do?"

One couple I know discovered the value of PLAY when they finally, after years of reluctance and resistance, scheduled a weekly date night.

Their resistance came from the sense that a scheduled time was too much pressure, too much expectation that "Now you *have* to have sex." Where was the desire? Where was the fun? Sex you had to schedule could never be sex worth having, because when they felt like they "had" to do something, they immediately did not want to do it.

But they had been struggling with infrequent sex, both wanting (in principle) to have sex more often but neither able to make it happen. They had tried so many things, and still they were stuck. So they considered scheduling a "sex night."

Then one of them had the brilliant idea that instead of "sex night," it was *game night*. They bought a set of those silly sex dice—and it turned out the silliness was what made the difference. Come game night, they alternated rolls of the dice.

One partner told me, "When we started, I thought the ritual would do what it hasn't done, which is 'prime the pump' so we'd have sex more often. But what it did was, during the most stressful times, times when one or both of us were just crawling-out-of-our-skin stressed, it kept us connected erotically even when anything else was just not going to happen."

No, they weren't having what they usually considered "sex" more often, but they were sharing pleasure, touching each other playfully and lovingly. That's one example of what centering pleasure, instead of desire, can look like. It can look like sustaining an erotic connection, even through the most stressful seasons of your lives, by playing together.

If it were up to me, almost all the sex in mainstream media would be full of giggling and laughter, jokes, wrestling, puns, and playing pretend. It would be like President and Dr. Bartlett on election night in season four of *The West Wing*, with the president half-ironically describing all the states he won and murmuring, "Who's your commander-in-chief?" and her answering in a breathy voice, "You are."

But almost no sex in the mainstream media is any damn fun. Why? Because play is, by definition, low-stakes, and anybody who writes stories knows you're supposed to keep the stakes high, to keep the audience engaged. Why watch people have zero-stakes, laughing sex, just for the fun of it?

Here's reason number 74 billion why sex in the media—mainstream or porn—is not like sex in real life. In real life, you want high stakes to be the exception, not the rule.

What are you doing when you experience the feeling of lightness, laughter, and friendship? When is your face relaxed and your attention almost effortlessly attuned to the present moment? What kind of play feels good to you? What kind of play feels good to your partner? What kind of play might make it feel easy to slide through the doorway into the sexytimes room?

For me, PLAY is jokes and silliness, rather than physical play. For a friend of mine, it's chasing, wrestling, and tickling. For some people, it's playful competition, for others it's playful collaboration. Which feels more friendship-building to you, playing against someone on an opposing team or playing with someone on the same team?

Another woman, on learning about the emotional floorplan, had this revelation: "On holiday, my partner and I fall so easily into this romantic, connected, playful space that makes it so easy to move into an erotic space. And I've always wondered, why is it so easy on holiday? Now I realize, oh! It's because we're in the PLAY space when we're on holiday!" (Her floorplan is the multistory townhome.) Couples' "getaways" are a common feature in people's narratives of when they have the most satisfying sex, perhaps especially for couples whose children are no longer little kids but are still very much in the house all the time.[6]

This isn't true for everyone, but it might be true for you. Is vacation PLAY?

As fictional interwar detective Lord Peter Wimsey says, "The only sin that passion can commit is to be joyless. It must lie down with laughter or makes its bed in hell; there can be no middle way." And on his wedding night, following a series of farcically unsexy fiascos, Lord Peter whispers to his chuckling bride as he climbs into bed, "What does it matter? What does anything matter? We are here. Laugh, lover, laugh. This is the end of the journey and the beginning of all delights."

As you consider the PLAY space in your emotional mind, you can ask yourself the same questions from the LUST section, but now you also begin to investigate the relationships among the different spaces:

- How do you know you're in that space?

- What happens in your body, thoughts, and emotions when you're there?

- How do you feel about this space?

- What spaces are adjacent?

- What pulls you into that space, and what pushes you out?

PLAY, WHEN THE STAKES ARE HIGH

I'm often asked by medical providers what couples can do to maintain a sexual connection while they're trying to get pregnant. My answer is simple: First, help them manage expectations, for example by being clear that it's not rare for it to take a year[7]—which can be inconvenient, I know. The couple may have a plan and a timeline, but their reproductive cells may or may not be on board.

And second: PLAY. Your partner is still a whole person, not just hormones and gametes, and you are still a whole person, too. Meet together in an erotic space that is for you as a couple, not for babymaking.

I began giving this advice to medical providers after I talked to a couple who waited in line for most of an hour to have a book signed and to tell me their story, hoping that I would tell others. They were among the many couples whose sex lives had been adversely affected by their efforts to get pregnant. Fertility treatment and the scheduling demands of planning sex around conception are notoriously damaging to the erotic connection between partners. After more than a year of this (which, again, is not rare), both AJ and her partner were burned out. They started resenting sex and each other.

When did things turn around for them?

When they decided it was funny.

They switched their mindset from dread, frustration, and self-doubt, to humor, play, and connection. It's a brilliant strategy, if you can manage it, though it isn't always easy. People's entire sense of self can be wrapped up in their efforts to become parents. Especially if there are pregnancy losses involved, the struggle can include profound grief. That's normal and real and nothing to make light of. And it's part of what makes this couple's story so important. They turned toward each other's difficult feelings with enough calm, warm curiosity to remember that, whether they got pregnant or not, they loved each other and wanted their partner to be happy. So they made it funny, for each other's sake.

Play is consequence-free, with zero stakes. For a lot of folks, that is the opposite of sex for conception. But sex is inherently funny, if you can see it through the emotional wall of wanting to get pregnant. I mean, when else in life is ejaculation so serious? Ejaculation, outside the context of fertilization, can be truly hilarious. Remember when ejaculation was fun and funny?

Inter-gamete couples (i.e., one person has sperm and one person has eggs) who expect to get pregnant by having intercourse have a very specific experience of how "trying" impacts your sex life. So, for inter-gamete reproducers of all genders: Remember PLAY. It is the antidote to the intensely high stakes that come with sex when you're trying to get pregnant.

SEEKING

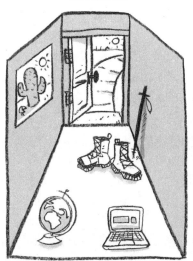

SEEKING is the space of exploration, curiosity, adventure, moving toward. What will you find, just beyond the door?

Also known by names like exploration, curiosity, adventure, or learning, SEEKING is the key to much of human endeavor, including our motivation to read a book about sex so that we can improve our lives. For some people, SEEKING can look like going to an art museum or seeing a movie or taking a cooking class or attending a lecture. It can be nerding out over a pop culture obsession, traveling to a foreign country, or meeting new people. Whether you're exploring with your body or with your mind or (most often) both, when you feel an urge to solve a problem, improve a system, have a new experience, or understand something you didn't before, you're in the SEEKING space. It's the "Oooooooooh, what's that?" state of mind that leads you to try something new.

SEEKING has always been my primary way in. All my relationships before my marriage happened while I was a student, and sexual initiation was easy because it flowed naturally from our ordinary conversation, which was often about my partner's research or mine. Shared intellectual exploration opened directly into LUST.

On the TV show *Grey's Anatomy*, season 13, episode 16, April and Jackson figure out how to do a never-before-attempted surgery together. Excitedly, they convince the guy in charge that this is a good idea, actually! They scrub in! They say "scalpel" at the same time! They operate together through sexy, affectionate eye gazing, made all the more intense by the fact that the only part of their faces we can see, between surgical masks and surgical caps, is their eyes . . . their shining, smiling eyes. They save a little girl's life *and* her voice! And what do they do when they get back to the hotel, exhausted from hours of surgery? Do they sleep? Heck no, not before they totally do it. Curiosity, exploration, problem-solving, high-stakes collaboration, all blend with their existing emotional and sexual connection, and they can't resist the pull into the LUST space.

If you have gotten to LUST through SEEKING, maybe you and your partner were solving problems together, whether it was a home plumbing DIY or an academic quandary. Or maybe you were traveling through unknown places and the adventure of it, the shared exploration, transformed into LUST when you got to bed that night.

LUST through SEEKING can also look like the couple I know who left their jobs, sold most of their stuff, and traveled together for a year. It was not always fun, but it was an *adventure*. Dwelling in a constant state of novelty, exploration, and shared problem-solving felt like foreplay, they said. Sounds exhausting to me, but I love it for them! They loved it for them, too, and they have the babies to show for it, which is still another adventure.

In what contexts do you experience curiosity? What do you love to learn about? What kinds of new experiences feel rewarding? What kinds of exploration are *not* interesting to you? Some people adore travel and all the novelty it brings, which might be a way into their LUST state. Some people would rather stay home, with the comfort and predictability it brings, which might be a way into their LUST state. People vary and they change, and there is no right or wrong. Get to know your sense of curiosity, because that space is going to be where a lot of problems get solved, as we'll see in part 2. Consider the questions:

- How do you know you're in SEEKING?

- What happens in your body, thoughts, and emotions when you're there?

- How do you feel about this space?

- What spaces are adjacent?

- What pulls you into that space, and what pushes you out?

CARE

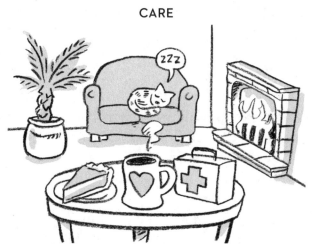

CARE is the space of love and tenderness, both "taking care of" and "caring for."

In *Come as You Are,* I called the CARE system by another of its scientific names, attachment, but its real-life name is simply love. It shows up deep in our biology, as in the burst of oxytocin that induces uterine contractions and mammary lactation at the end of pregnancy. To care and be cared for is a biological drive; humans sicken and even die from loneliness.

If what you want when you want sex is connection, you're linking CARE and LUST. For some people, sex is a fairly peripheral expression of CARE, but for others, perhaps especially those with reliably higher sexual desire, sex may be the most powerful way of being in CARE.

Because it's such a sprawling part of the human experience, I like to think of CARE as an open-concept room, with multiple functional areas all in one big space. The "living room" of CARE has a cozy fireplace, a cushy sofa, and a soft rug to dig your toes into. It's the room in which adults exist in a loving, mutually supportive peer relationship full of affection and joy and trust and admiration. For a lot of people there's a hallway or even just a door straight from the living room of CARE into the garden of LUST.

One of my favorite fictional examples of living room, "caring for" CARE in a romance novel is Alyssa Cole's *Radio Silence*. When suddenly there is no power, no cellphones, no running water, and no one knows why, Arden and Gabriel depend on each other to survive, even though they don't like each other much at first. Through their struggles to stay alive, they build a bond of intimacy. It's not one person taking care of the other, but mutual care, mutual responsibility. When they overreact emotionally—which of course they do sometimes, because *it's an apocalypse*—they apologize. When they have any opportunity to think beyond food and shelter and injuries, they consider each other's comfort and pleasure— baths, music, and, above all, creating moments of kindness to hold each other's grief. As their situation stabilizes and their connection grows stronger, they learn to comfort each other, reading aloud from a stash of romance novels they find in a cabin, or, as Arden puts it, fucking each other senseless. That's how "caring for" can connect to the LUST room.

But our open-concept room of CARE also has a kitchen, where you "take care of" rather than "care for" others. This is the workhorse of the CARE room. It's powerful and beautiful, but if you're taking care of your partner in the kitchen of CARE, it can feel too much like parenting, and it does not lead straight to the bedroom. When CARE shows up as "cleaning up after," that's rarely sexy.

Many parents of small children are in a state of constant near-panic and exhaustion. Their lives consist of endless laundry, dishes, schedules of pickups and drop-offs, crackers and juice boxes. Even when a couple is collaborating effectively, working as a team to meet their family's needs, they're often stuck in an emotional corner, unable to get to LUST or PLAY or SEEKING. Nan Wise, in her book *Why Good Sex Matters,* describes this to a client in her own inimitable way: "Your CARE system is cockblocking your LUST system!"

And it can be even worse when one partner isn't just taking care of the small young humans in their home; if they're also caretaking for the other partner, it's an emotional hall of mirrors. You're in CARE and everything you look at is CARE—meaning a responsibility, an obligation, a requirement, a duty to sacrifice your time, energy, and emotion in the service of these other people. Of course you can't get to LUST from there!

If getting stuck in the caretaking corner is your situation, the language of the dual nature of the CARE space can help you talk with your partner about how to get out.

Your partner can say, "I see you're trapped in CARE, I hear you saying that even loving touch is irritating because it only feels like more kid hands touching you. What help do you need, so that you can get out of CARE and get some rest?"

In a heterosexual relationship, the humorous term "choreplay" comes from the idea that women get turned on seeing their husbands do chores. It's why I always get a laugh when I say, "Sometimes the sexiest thing you can do . . . is the dishes." A friend of mine once told me, "Forget roses. When it's fifteen degrees [Fahrenheit] out and the wind is howling and my husband is under the car hood trying to get it started so you can go somewhere, *that* opens the door to the LUST room." Choreplay is caring for, which can help a partner escape the caretaking corner.

When therapist Esther Perel talks about intimacy as an enemy of passion, CARE is what she's talking about. But when John Gottman talks about intimacy as a key to passion, it's what he's talking about, too. She means the caretaking corner; he means the living room of "caring for."

As you consider the CARE space in your emotional mind, ask yourself the questions:

- How do you know you're in that space?

- What happens in your body, thoughts, and emotions when you're there?

- How do you feel about this space?

- What spaces are adjacent?

- What pulls you into that space, and what pushes you out?

Ama and Di

Romantic comedies, for all their faults, can illustrate how PLAY creates an erotic context. Take my friend Ama. A mom and wife with a full-time job plus a side hustle, she gets one night each week entirely to herself, while her wife, Di, takes care of their three kids, who range in age from toddler to teenager. What does she choose to do with this time alone? Exercise? Pray? Nap? Any of the other activities she knows nourish her? No, she can do all of that in her daily life; this is not a time for nourishment, it's a time for indulgence. In this protected downtime, Ama watches rom-coms.

Ama and Di already communicated well about sex, but the metaphor of the floorplan offered language to articulate something Ama had noticed but not been able to describe. After Ama learned about the emotional floorplan, she told me how it helped her express her observation and how she and Di put it into action:

"I was watching this rom-com and I noticed these char-

acters were hardcore teasing each other and that's what was hot about their connection. And I realized that's what I want! A PLAY approach to connection. I want humor and levity, which we have very little of in our lives right now just because we have so much life management with work and the kids and everything."

As the lower-desire partner (even in a strong, satisfied sexual connection, there may be a partner with lower desire) with a stressful, exhausting life, Ama wanted to find more ways into erotic connection. Having the language of the room next door helped her communicate this idea to her partner.

"We had both had a long day, but Di joined me in the shower, which is a place where we can just talk about things, and she asked what I was thinking about. I said, 'I think I need joking around.' Before I might have said something like 'I need you to be happy,' which is an unreasonable thing to ask, obviously. Like, a person can't just be happy. But she can play around.

"And she did, all that next day, teasing me and joking with me, being playful, and that night we had the most amazing sex!"

(Ama's floorplan, below, is based on a traditional Asante building, inspired by her Ghanaian heritage.)

I want to point out an especially insightful aspect of Ama's new language. She transitioned from "I need you to be happy" to "I need joking around." That's a transition from "I need your individual internal state to change" to "I need our shared dynamic to change." In other words, "It's not your job, it's our shared job."

For anyone who wants their partner to want them spontaneously, like Mike, or wants themselves to want sex more easily, like Margot, this is how you transition away from wanting to change someone (yourself or someone else) toward wanting to change the context.

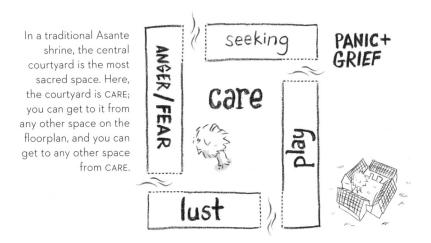

In a traditional Asante shrine, the central courtyard is the most sacred space. Here, the courtyard is CARE; you can get to it from any other space on the floorplan, and you can get to any other space from CARE.

The Pleasure-Adverse Spaces

And now we come to the "adverse" emotional spaces—that is, the spaces that we're motivated to avoid experiencing. PANIC/GRIEF, FEAR, and RAGE are distinct from one another, but they are all emotional spaces where we are likely to interpret sensations as potential threats, things to be avoided.

As you read, remember this:

Difficult feelings are not dangerous.

Difficult feelings are not dangerous because they, like all feelings, are tunnels. When you go all the way through them, you get to the light at the end. They may be uncomfortable, for sure; that's kind of their point. When you experience them, that's your embodied mind alerting you that it perceives a potential problem or a threat. But the feelings themselves are not dangerous, just as a lifeguard's whistle alerting everyone to get out of the ocean is not dangerous. What's potentially dangerous is the shark or the rip current or the lightning; that's why you get out of the water. There is no need to fear the whistle.

Most of the time, these three emotional spaces are distant from LUST. But, because difficult, pleasure-adverse emotions are inevitable in any relationship that lasts long enough, getting to know these spaces is essential to learning to cultivate a sexual connection over many years.

PANIC/GRIEF

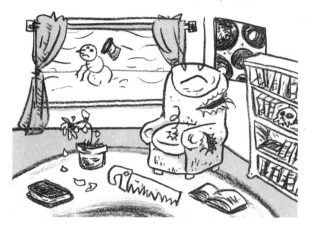

PANIC/GRIEF is the space of lost connection, loneliness, and abandonment. Because love is a biological drive—meaning we can die if we don't get enough—this space is an alert system to tell us when we're feeling too alone. PANIC is the warning of isolation; GRIEF is feeling helpless and hopeless.

PANIC/GRIEF is directly connected to whether or not we are receiving enough CARE. At its simplest, PANIC/GRIEF is loneliness. But loneliness is like hunger; it's an alarm sounding, telling us to fix a problem that could lead to serious harm.

You see, a human infant's life literally depends on their adult caregivers, so our brains have a powerful PANIC/GRIEF warning system that alerts us that bad things could happen if no one comes to us when we need help. The absence of a caregiver activates PANIC in young humans—tears and wailing and efforts to find or engage with the caregiver. If the caregiver still doesn't come back, behavior transitions into the GRIEF half of PANIC/GRIEF—sadness and, if the isolation goes on too long, eventually hopeless despair.

Around adolescence, the CARE system gets co-opted and our peers become our attachment objects. By adulthood, our lives no longer literally depend on our attachment object coming back, but our bodies don't know that. So separation from a lover can feel like you're dying. They call it heartbreak for a reason.

Like all these primary emotional spaces, PANIC/GRIEF has a range of intensities that modulate how easy it is to move from there to LUST. At lower intensities, PANIC/GRIEF can fuel many different kinds of LUSTful experiences. Jessamyn Stanley, a polyamorous queer yoga teacher, said on her podcast, "Jealousy is my kink."[8] When her nestmate was developing a relationship with a new partner, it activated a low-level sense of threat to the attachment, a tension that in turn activates LUST as a way to reinforce the bond in their relationship.

Sometimes, breakups and major arguments can also catapult us from PANIC/GRIEF to LUST. When our connection with the other person is destabilized, our brains will harness every tool they have to stabilize the connection. Sex is one of the ways we stabilize, reinforce, and even restore connection with our peers. Hence breakup sex and makeup sex. The stakes of breakup and makeup sex may feel life-threateningly high; hence all the breakup and makeup sex in soap operas, movies, and romance novels. These stories construct sexual touch almost exclusively as a way to ease PANIC/GRIEF. No one ever feels actual pleasure or joy, just relief. I want more for your sex life than relief from existential despair. I want joy for you.

But for some people, the least hint of jealousy or discord can lock the door to LUST. A friend of mine with a significant history of abusive relationships told me that it has taken him a long time to learn that it's okay when his partner spends time with other people. For most of his life, if a partner expressed any admiration for someone else, his brain just assumed the relationship was over, his partner was going to leave him for this other person, and so rather than panicking and trying to repair the relationship, his body would shut down and disengage completely.

As you consider the PANIC/GRIEF space in your emotional mind, ask yourself the questions:

- How do you know you're in that space?

- What happens in your body, thoughts, and emotions when you're there?

- How do you feel about this space?

- What spaces are adjacent?

- What pushes you into that space, and what pulls you out? (Notice that this is different from the first four spaces. In general, we are *pulled* into the positive emotions and *pushed* into the negative emotions.)

FEAR

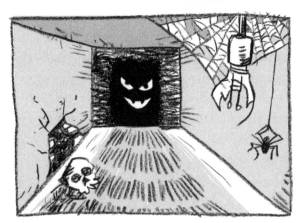

FEAR is the space of "Unsafe! Move away!" At its lowest intensity, it might be a slight niggling worry; at higher intensities it can be full terror. It can also show up as people-pleasing, doing whatever it takes to create a sense of safety.

In everyday language, FEAR is everything from a slight worry to anxiety to terror. FEAR is amazing, because it could be three different things: flight, fawn, and freeze—not fight; fight is RAGE, which we'll talk about next.

FEAR's classic outward manifestation is flight, a "chaotic projectile movement to get out of harm's way," according to Jaak Panksepp. Evolutionarily, FEAR is there to help us survive life-threatening situations like being chased by a predator, and when you're being chased by something with teeth and claws that can run thirty miles per hour and wants to eat you, there is no need for curiosity or sex. What you need is to *survive*. So FEAR may also include "reduced positive affect," that is, an inhibition of the favorable systems of PLAY, SEEKING, CARE, and LUST.

Or it can show up as something sometimes called "fawn" or "tend and befriend"—a highly social threat response that causes us to seek connection as a way of finding safety. We smile and placate a dangerous-seeming person, especially those with power over us. We protect and take care of the vulnerable people around us to try to make them safe in an unsafe situation. We look to the faces of the people around us, seeking reassurance that we're not alone in this threatening situation. We run to someone safe and hold on hard to them. This version of FEAR may involve the CARE system, but it's in the kitchen of CARE, with a hot stove covered in pots filled with boiling oil and you can't look away for a second, for fear of fire.

But FEAR can also show up as "freeze," where you shut down, collapse, long for sleep, can't speak or think clearly, can barely move, or feel that you're in a fog, moving in slow motion. Freeze is our last-ditch FEAR response, when your brain has lost hope that you can escape the threat or defeat the threat or persuade the threat to go away. Sometimes people talk about it as "going into shock" or "playing dead." Physiologically, your brain and body are waiting for the threat to pass or for help to come. Given that a significant proportion of people have experienced sexual trauma, often including the experience of freeze, it's not rare for LUST to have a one-way doorway directly into FEAR.

Here's one example of getting stuck in FEAR, when you want to get to LUST. (If you're a survivor of sexual violence, you may prefer to skip to the end of this section.) A young woman experienced a traumatic groping, where a man approached her from behind and grabbed her genitals with his hand and pressed his genitals against her back. This was in public, in a store, in full daylight. This guy just grabbed her and groped her and then walked away. She never even saw his face. Her body shut down, going straight to freeze. In a haze, she left the store, made her way home, and got into bed, hiding under the covers, and waited until she was able to cry. Then she did her best to forget about it.

Years later, she was in a relationship and happy. She and her partner moved in together, and things were going well. Then one day, as she was standing at the sink washing dishes, her partner came home and wrapped his arms around her—from behind. Her body freaked out. Her arms went in front of her face and her body froze, trembling with tension.

The past incident had created a trapdoor in her brain, so that when her partner approached her from behind, she fell helplessly into FEAR. And the only path out of the FEAR went through RAGE. She became angry with herself for being "irrational," then she was angry with her partner for surprising her that way, then she was angry at her groper for creating this emotional trap in her brain. But mostly she was just angry and looking for a target, and there wasn't one, and so she got stuck.

Worst of all, that trapdoor expanded and generalized to other sexual touch, whether being held from behind or not. Eventually almost any sexual touch would send her down through the trapdoor into FEAR.

What did they do?

Well, they talked about it. They made a plan to try safe, controlled touch together, and gradually, over weeks, increase the intimacy of their shared touch, teaching her body that sexual touch can happen in a safe-enough context. Just as the trapdoor into fear could grow, it could also be shrunk, by practicing touch in the context of safety.

Do I have to mention they worked with a therapist?

If you or a partner are a survivor of sexual violence, there may be nothing more powerful than exploring how your brain has linked LUST and FEAR, based on your life experience, and gently allowing your brain to learn to experience sexual stimulation *in the context of safety.* Training your brain to unlink FEAR and LUST takes time and love, like training a puppy; if you get frustrated or impatient, you only make the puppy feel shy and worried. Your FEARful brain is like that puppy. Treat it with love, patience, and appreciation for how hard it's trying to do things right, and it will learn that it is safe. It will relax and blossom.

A necessary caveat about FEAR: If your fear derives not from past experiences or worries about the future, but from your current partner, that's a sign that something very serious is going wrong in your relationship. If you're afraid of your partner, if your partner shames you for your fear, if you get into a FEAR space and can't find a way out: therapy. Those are bigger, more fundamental problems than a book can help you with.

FEAR is a part of life. The goal is not to live without FEAR, but to live with it in ways that let you move through it, rather than allowing it to decide what you do or don't do in your life.

Audre Lorde offered poetic wisdom about living with fear in her *Cancer Journals*. She wrote:

> *"I am learning to live beyond fear by living through it, and in the process learning to turn fury at my own limitations into some more creative energy. . . . If I cannot banish fear completely I can learn to count with it less. For then fear becomes not a tyrant against which I waste my energy fighting, but a companion, not particularly desirable, yet one whose knowledge can be useful."*

If fear is a regular part of your life, let it become a useful companion, however unpleasant. As you consider the FEAR space in your emotional mind, ask yourself the questions:

- How do you know you're in that space?

- What happens in your body, thoughts, and emotions when you're there?

- How do you feel about this space?

- What spaces are adjacent?

- What pushes you into that space, and what pulls you out?

DEPRESSION AND ANXIETY
AND THE EMOTIONAL FLOORPLAN

If anxiety is or has been a part of your life, as it has been a part of mine, you'll recognize the physical, mental, or emotional turmoil of an ungrounded urge to escape, avoid, or chaotically attempt to control your environment. Whether you experience social anxiety, phobias, obsessive or compulsive behaviors or thoughts (such as disordered eating, picking at your skin or pulling out your hair, or counting, tapping, or checking things like locked doors, etc.), general anxiety, or all of these, anxiety is your body's way of trying to keep you safe in situations it has been trained to perceive as unsafe. Learning to notice when you're in the FEAR space and to ease your body through and out of it is the essential skill of reducing the impact of anxiety on your life. And, of course, reducing the impact of anxiety on your life can only increase your brain's access to pleasure and LUST.

Similarly, PANIC/GRIEF is where depression lives, and for most people, the intensity of PANIC/GRIEF is an emotional swamp, making it difficult to get to any favorable spaces, including LUST. If depression is or has been a part of your life, as it has been a part of mine, you may be familiar with the shadows of helplessness and isolation that seem to follow you around in this space. This is why many of the effective treatments for depression involve bodily autonomy and social connection, especially PLAY. Physical activity teaches your body that you are not trapped and helpless, whatever your brain's opinion might be. Connection with others teaches you that you are not alone and, thus, that you do not in fact deserve to be alone. Learning to notice when you're in the PANIC/GRIEF space and to ease your body through and out of it is the essential skill of reducing the impact of depression on your life. In chapter 5 you'll find the relationship skills that facilitate working as a team.

RAGE

Known in everyday language by names like anger, annoyance, irritation, frustration, or sometimes hatred, RAGE is the "attack mode" of the stress response. It is a biological impulse to *move toward and destroy* something we perceive as a threat to our safety, well-being, identity, or goals.

What are some things that activate RAGE inside you? What causes hate to rise, making you want to destroy or wish something or someone would cease to exist?

RAGE is the space of "Unsafe! Move to destroy!" It can be as small as annoyance or irritation and as large as a body-filling Hulk-like need to smash. No emotion is inherently dangerous, but because RAGE is the motivation to break things, we have to be sure we don't trust our hands or our words when RAGE is intensely activated.

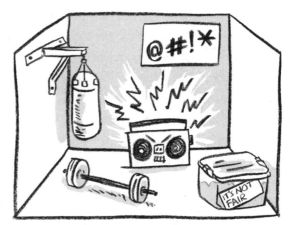

Of all the rooms in your emotional floorplan, RAGE is the room people have the most complicated feelings about. It's a space many of us have been taught we don't or shouldn't have. And if you can't recognize that you're in RAGE, that makes it pretty difficult to get out.

My general advice for addressing intense anger in a relationship is: When you're deep in the RAGE room, no touching each other, not with any part of your body. Also, no words. You can growl and pound on your chest like a gorilla. You can jump up and down or go for a run or emit a primal scream with your partner, to purge the rage from your body. Feelings are tunnels; you have to go through them to get to the light. But no words and no touching, not even directed toward yourself.

Your anger is not inherently harmful, and if you don't use your body or words as weapons, the mere existence of your anger is not dangerous. Nor is your partner's anger inherently harmful, and if they do not use their body or words as weapons, the mere existence of their anger is not dangerous. You can be angry in each other's presence, you can even be angry with each other, and *nothing is wrong*.

Another necessary caveat, like the one for FEAR: If your partner uses their rage to excuse using their body or words as a weapon against you, or if you allow yourself to cause harm to your partner because you "lost your temper," something seriously not okay is happening. Seek professional intervention.

What *can* we do in the RAGE space? We purge. We throw stuff into trash bags and out the metaphorical window, we allow the tide of the emotion to flood through us and to dissipate. We do not tie the physiology of our emotion to any thoughts or ideas; we don't believe anything we tell ourselves (it's not possible to distinguish between truth and self-serving lies in the RAGE room). We pull weeds from the metaphorical garden.

A friend of mine had gotten as far as acknowledging that she had a RAGE space in her emotional floorplan; she could even recognize that she was in it. What my friend asked, though, was not how to deal with RAGE. It was "How am I supposed to want sex, when I have all this rage?"

At first, I didn't understand the question. I asked her to explain, and she described all her frustration from years of feeling "like a subordinate," she said. It was a role she was raised to believe was her duty, but after decades of marriage, she had grown more and more disillusioned with those beliefs and more and more frustrated as her husband made no space for her to pursue her own dreams, as he failed to accept more responsibility for day-to-day household-ing and helping with the kids, now in their teens, and as he mini-mized her distress and told her she was just better at these things. And why was she angry? That was a compliment! Over time, her rage had accumulated and calcified into a wall of contempt.

She asked again, "How do I want sex, in the midst of all this?"

"Well . . . first of all," I said, "it's not desire that matters, it's pleasure. But you don't have to want or like sex all the time. You don't have to keep trying to get to LUST, you can just focus on get-ting through RAGE." There's no reason to want or like sex if you're spending a lot of time in the RAGE space.

With that said, we are often taught that RAGE and LUST are closely linked and maybe even belong together. It's a lie, but it's so ubiquitous that it's only natural that you would believe it. We grow up accepting the (neurologically silly) notion that wanting to approach someone to destroy them must be very similar to wanting to approach someone to share an erotic experience. It shows up in pop culture all the time—side-eye to the 2005 *Pride & Prejudice,* in which Darcy and Lizzy almost kiss immediately after she explains to him all the ways she hates him.[9]

In RAGE-motivated LUST, you want to fuck someone as a way to destroy them. But that's not sex, that's sexual violence—using sex as a weapon against someone. And a blanket *no* to that. Never try to destroy someone with sex, without their full, free consent. We all get that, right? It's the twenty-first century; we understand that using sex to hurt, punish, or destroy someone is always, always bad, right? Okay, good.

Are there times when RAGE and LUST can co-exist? Sure, I can think of at least two.

First, some breakup sex and makeup sex may fall into this category, though I think PANIC/GRIEF is more usual. When there's an argument in an established relationship and the conflict creates a threat to the attachment bond, humans use sex as an attachment behavior, to reinforce and heal damage to attachment. These kinds of experiences blend CARE with RAGE and LUST.

A second possibility involves one partner happily consenting to being "destroyed" with sex, while another person happily consents to do it. It's nearly always *metaphorical* destruction and highly stylized rage. These kinds of experiences blend PLAY with RAGE and LUST. It calls for exceptionally good communication skills, so you can stay clear about boundaries even during intense emotional experiences. This kind of play nearly always happens in a preexisting relationship grounded in trust.

Whether through CARE or PLAY, skilled partners integrate RAGE with LUST by choosing a shared target for their rage. They don't want to destroy their partner, they want to destroy, say, a person who did them harm in the past or a subject of conflict in the relationship or an unchosen, unwanted part of themselves. They may play pretend, acting like one of them is the person who did harm, but the partner is never the literal target of RAGE.

Please, let's retire the "angry sex" narrative and replace it with playful sex. So much better for all of us! Wanting to destroy someone and wanting to connect erotically are not related, except under specific, fairly extraordinary circumstances.

RAGE has a place in our lives and in our relationships and even in our eroticism. It is an important and wholesome dimension of our internal lives. But it's complicated because it is the biology of destruction, domination, and control. It's also complicated because our relationship to our own and other people's anger has been shaped our whole lives by cultural messages, as I'll discuss in the coming chapters. But for now, the moral of the story is: When we are in the RAGE space, no hands, no words. Don't go into LUST from RAGE unless you and your partner are making mutual and intentional choices. Never engage sexually with someone you feel an impulse to destroy.

As you consider the RAGE space in your emotional mind, ask yourself the questions:

- How do you know you're in that space?

- What happens in your body, thoughts, and emotions when you're there?

- How do you feel about this space?

- What spaces are adjacent?

- What pushes you into that space, and what pulls you out?

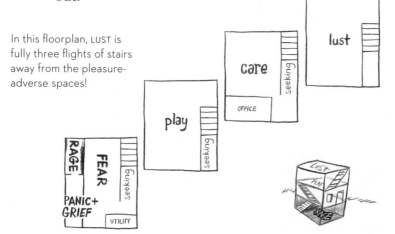

In this floorplan, LUST is fully three flights of stairs away from the pleasure-adverse spaces!

Two Bonus Spaces

In addition to the seven primary process emotions, as outlined by Jaak Panksepp, I want to add two further spaces in your floorplan. These are not emotions, but they are crucial influences on our sexualities and our relationships, and they deserve space on a floorplan that explores where you might be relative to your LUST space.

THE FIRST BONUS SPACE IS YOUR THINKING MIND. I often imagine the THINKING MIND as an office, where your thinking, planning, worrying, ruminating, cognition, and social appropriateness live. It's where people get stuck when they can't "get out of their heads." They can't disengage from the past or the future in order to be present with their partner and their body's sensations. We "moderns," as Buddhist teacher Sebene Selassie calls us, are prone to this kind of stuckness, living in our heads as if our minds were just bubbles, floating, disconnected, above our bodies.

And it's where a lot of us get stuck, when we're trying to get to LUST.

The specific nature of your office will vary depending on a lot of factors. A woman with ADHD said, "I suspect mine is actually huge and chaotic. I see it as a room filled with precariously stacked boxes that are blocking the access to rooms in my brain." A man with autism said, "I think my office is my favorite place inside my head, and inside my head is my favorite place in the world, so it's a lot of work to drag my attention away from a space full of my favorite toys and go spend time somewhere else."

As you consider your THINKING MIND all the same questions apply:

- How do you know you're in this space?

- What happens in your body, thoughts, and emotions when you're in there?

- How do you feel about your thinking mind?

- What spaces are adjacent to it?

- What pushes or pulls you into it, and what takes you out?

THE UTILITY ROOM

In addition to all the thoughts and emotions that together make you you, you also have a body, and that body has needs, like for food and water and sleep and love. It communicates those needs up to the brain, so that the brain can figure out how to get those needs met. I think of the meet-basic-needs brain processes as a UTILITY ROOM. In a house, this might be the place where the plumbing and heating and bathroom fixtures and other necessary infrastructure are tucked away. In your brain, it's your need for air, water, food, sleep, and all the physiological necessities of life. Every single one of these needs takes priority over sex. If you are ill, exhausted, or hungry, those are all legitimate, brakes-hitting contextual factors that reduce your brain's access to pleasure. We spend our lives checking in on the UTILITY ROOM, so that our needs can be met.

THE SECOND BONUS SPACE IS OBSERVATIONAL DISTANCE. It is also known by names like "mindfulness," "Self," "decentering," or "self-as-context."[10] Going there is the skill of stepping to one side of your internal experience so that you can observe it without being *in* it. Mindfulness teachers often describe it as a kind of scenic viewpoint, like you find on hiking trails in national parks or along mountain roads. From a distance, we can notice what's happening in our bodies and minds, without having an opinion about it or trying to change anything.

"Notice without trying to change" is the key here. Throughout the book, we'll talk about how to create change, and it will almost always involve spending some time at the scenic viewpoint, neutrally noticing our internal experience. We're going to rely on our ability to notice what's happening, to understand and appreciate the ways our minds and bodies are trying to keep us safe and satisfied, before we try to change anything. My personal experience of OBSERVATIONAL DISTANCE is so important that I consider it my emotional "home base," where I return whenever I want to feel safe inside my own internal experience.

If you've tried mindfulness before and hated it, never fear. Any practice that involves witnessing our internal experience, as an outside observer, without being "in it," takes us to the scenic viewpoint. Sure, when we practice sitting meditation or yoga or tai chi or mindful breathing, we practice going to the scenic viewpoint. But some people get to this space of OBSERVATIONAL DISTANCE when they exercise. Others get there when they knit. Some get there through music, dance, art. I mostly get there by writing. My spouse gets there by doing something that's just a little bit engaging—mowing the lawn, getting groceries, mindless little games on his handheld game console—and allowing the rest of his mind to wander. If you already know what gets you to the scenic viewpoint, I recommend making whatever it is a regular practice. If you don't yet know what gets you there, begin with an appealing form of rhythmic movement, whether it's yoga, tai chi, Feldenkrais, or dance of any kind, all of which are adaptable to different abilities.[11] If movement is not for you, try a formal mindfulness practice of sitting or lying down, while breathing and practicing nonjudgmental awareness of your thoughts.

As you consider your OBSERVATIONAL DISTANCE, all the same questions apply:

- How do you know you're in this space?

- What happens in your body, thoughts, and emotions when you're in there?

- How do you feel about your observational distance?

- What spaces are adjacent to it?

- What pushes or pulls you into it, and what takes you out?

Nine rooms is a big house. In a house that size, there are bound to be spaces you can't get to without going through some other room, the way you often can't get to the kitchen directly from the bedroom; you have to go through the living room or the dining room or maybe both. If all of your biological drives and primary process emotions are spaces in your mental house, the LUST room is a room you can't get to directly from every room—you have to go through some other room. The purpose of drawing your own emotional floorplan is to figure out which rooms in your house are next door to LUST and how to navigate out of the rooms that are far away from LUST. When you are stuck in the RAGE space, how can you find your way to LUST? Maybe it's through the living room of CARE or maybe it's through PLAY? You'll have to figure out what works for you. There is no right answer—every individual's floorplan will look different.

Now that you have an understanding of each "room," try drawing your own floorplan.

In the next chapter, I show you how to use it.

TIPS FOR STARTING YOUR FLOORPLAN

If you're not sure how to start exploring your own floorplan, here are some ideas you might try:

o On a blank sheet of paper, write the word LUST in the middle and then write the other spaces close to or far away from it on the page. These simple clusters will give you a rough idea of where to start.

o Alternatively, begin with the space where you feel like you spend the most time. From there, identify what spaces you tend to move into from that space.

Tend to oscillate between CARE and FEAR? What draws you out of either of those spaces, and where do you go from each? If you're not sure, it can help to identify spaces where you definitely don't go—for example if you never transition from FEAR directly into LUST, that's helpful information.

o Get to know each space individually, especially if you're struggling to understand how it fits into your emotional floorplan. Consider:

☐ Names of the different emotions that happen in that space—e.g., for RAGE you might have irritation, annoyance, frustration, and impatience, as well as anger, hatred, and rage itself; or for PLAY you might have lightheartedness, laughter, ease, friendship, connection, or cheering someone on.

☐ Adjectives that describe what it feels like to be in this space—tight or loose, warm or cold, free or trapped, and so on.

☐ Objects that would be in this space, if it were a literal room in a home—maybe a punching bag in the RAGE space, a bathtub in the CARE space, or a ceaseless rain in the PANIC/GRIEF space.

☐ A memory of a time when you were in this space, including what put you into it, how it felt to be there, and what moved you out of it. *What space did you move into?* The answer to that last question tells you if spaces might be close together.

o This process of exploring your floorplan is itself
practice at being in OBSERVATIONAL DISTANCE. As
you go through this process, notice when it's easy to
stay outside of the spaces you're considering and
when you get drawn into them, feeling the feelings
and thinking the thoughts of the space, instead of
observing the feelings and noticing the thoughts
of the space. Putting the feelings and thoughts on
paper (or typing on a screen) can help you strengthen
your skill at shifting to the scenic viewpoint.

Chapter 3 tl;dr:

- Our emotional brains have pleasure-favorable spaces—
LUST, PLAY, SEEKING, and CARE—and pleasure-adverse
spaces—PANIC/GRIEF, FEAR, and RAGE. Beyond those
emotional spaces, we also have our THINKING MINDS,
our bodies, and OBSERVATIONAL DISTANCE, the wise,
mindful practice of being able to step to one side to
witness our internal experience.

- It is essential for couples in a long-term sexual connection to understand their emotional spaces—
knowing how to recognize which space they're in,
what moves them into each one, what moves them
out, and how they feel about each space.

- It's also valuable to understand the relationships
among the various emotional spaces. Which are adjacent to each other? Which require a great deal of
change in order to transition from one to another?

- For couples who like the sex available to them but feel
"stuck" and unable to access the LUST space, learning

to get to the spaces adjacent to LUST can make it easier to move into LUST.

Some Good Questions:

- For each of the pleasure-favorable spaces: How do I know I'm in it? What does it feel like? What pulls me into it? What might push me out?

- For each of the pleasure-adverse spaces: How do I know I'm in it? What does it feel like? What pushes me into it? What might pull me out?

- How can I tell which space my partner might be in? What helps transition my partner from an adverse space to a pleasurable one? How do I feel about each of their pleasure-favorable and pleasure-adverse spaces?

- What are some effective ways my partners and I can communicate to each other what space we are in and what might help us transition to a different one? Can we be present for our partners' difficult feelings, and can our partners be present for our own?

Chapter 4

HOW TO USE YOUR FLOORPLAN;

or, Finding the Room Next Door to the Room Where It Happens

The point of understanding all these emotional spaces and how they're related to one another is to learn how to become unstuck and to help a partner become unstuck. Now that you've drawn your emotional floorplan, let's put it to work—first, by aiming for a space adjacent to LUST rather than for LUST itself, and, second, by engaging with your own and your partner's floorplan as "third things." You are not turning toward each other directly, you are turning your mutual gaze on these representations of your inner worlds.

Don't get too hung up on the idea of a literal floorplan. Doorways can be magical, with hidden passages and chutes that carry you from one space to another without anyone seeing how you did it. A door you can walk through in one direction may lock behind you, so you have to exit another way. This is not a literal floorplan; it has secrets and a life of its own, because it is *you*.

Aim for the "Room Next Door" to LUST

When I considered my emotional floorplan, I had an insight. I realized that when I tried to go directly from wherever I was to the LUST space, I inevitably got lost. What worked better was to aim not for LUST itself, but for a space that has a way in to LUST. I didn't need to find my way to the sexy space; I only needed to find my way to a mental space that was *adjacent* to the sexy space. So, in this chapter, we are on a search for your room next door to "the room where it happens."

What is your way in to LUST? What is your room next door to the room where it happens? Trace the paths from where you are to where you want to be. Which spaces connect to LUST? And what helps you to move out of any given space into a different one? These are the crucial questions when you're struggling to make your way to the LUST space.

For example, if you're in RAGE, irritated or even enraged with your partner, you almost certainly can't get directly from there to LUST. You probably don't even *want* to get to LUST. But you can figure out a path from RAGE to CARE, which might eventually lead you to LUST.

Maybe your floorplan is like that of an artist friend of mine, whose way in is through drawing their partner. The act of figure drawing shifts their attention into a mode that isn't itself erotic, but it's adjacent to the erotic; it's precise and focused and appreciative, searching for the uniqueness and thus the beauty of the body they're drawing. This is their version of SEEKING → LUST.

Maybe your path is like that of a different friend of mine, who is a parent of little kids. Watching her partner care for their kids is certainly not erotic, but it takes her to an emotional place in her brain, a place of gratitude and admiration, that is much closer to sexy than her "Mommy mode." This is her version of CARE → LUST.

People vary, and they change across their lifespans, and they're all normal.

What I Did

I'm going to tell the story of my own search for a new way in, but the moral of the story is not "Do what I did." It's "This simple idea turned out to be difficult, but also made me a better human and a better wife, plus it improved my sex life!" You may find the process easier than I did, but I don't want to candy-coat it like it's a breeze. Some sexual difficulties have their roots in our childhood bullshit and can't be fixed with tips or tricks or even a good metaphor or a story about someone else's way forward.

When I was struggling with desire, I tried asking myself different questions. Sex therapist Gina Ogden would suggest people complete the statement "I turn myself on when . . ." and Esther Perel does, too. If that prompt elicits great information for you, awesome. Use it. But it never elicited anything in me beyond ". . . when I masturbate?"

My turn-ons dwell exclusively in a space of *connection with another mind,* even if that mind is the author of some erotica I'm reading or it's a mind I made up in a fantasy. So that really good question didn't happen to be a good fit for me.

But then I thought about the emotional spaces in my mind and I asked myself: What is my "way in" to an erotic state of mind?

This is when I realized that SEEKING was my primary way in—and SEEKING wasn't working. Everyone I've ever been in love with has been someone whose mind I admired and wanted to explore and learn from. My partner now is no exception—but his mind is different. He's not a scientist or any kind of academic. He's an artist. He thinks in images and spatial relationships, which are my weakest ways of understanding the world. I think in words and human dynamics, so the sociologist, the cognitive scientist, the philosopher, the other philosopher, even the film studies person, they were natural fits with the way my mind works. With all of them, my way into erotic connection was through SEEKING: my intellect, my curiosity, my "social science" brain. But with my spouse, that can't be my primary way into erotic connection, because that's not a space where he spends a lot of time.

He lives in lots of other spaces where I don't spend a lot of time. Art and design. Writing jokes. Those are fun places to go with him, but they are not adjacent to the LUST room in my mind.

There was a time when I wondered if our erotic connection would work, because we couldn't spend much time together in my delightful world of affective neuroscience, parsing precise distinctions between important concepts. Early in our relationship I tried to connect with him through science, and I just ended up frustrated because he would make jokes, because that's what he does to connect. Neither of us was aware that I was trying to build an erotic connection by talking about science, so neither of us understood why I got so frustrated and felt so lonely because of it.

But in all those previous loves, where I had entered into the erotic through the intellect, the intellectual connection was solid and the physical connection was solid, but the emotional connection was . . . a mess. The mess of those shared emotional connections is why all those relationships ended.

With my spouse, the emotional connection is *buh-na-naaaaaaaahhhhzzzzz*. He's so thoroughly there for me. All my decades of practice masking my feelings are nothing to him, he sees right through the mask. He sees me and loves me. He even understands why I need the mask. For all this and more, my emotional connection with him is unlike anything I've experienced with anyone else, and he is stuck with me forever because of it. Sorry, dude, if you were expecting to marry somebody else someday, you should not have been so loving and supportive.

But. No matter how amazing our emotional connection is, that was never my way into erotic connection. In fact, it was strangely distant from erotic connection; his emotional intelligence, his ability to read my state of mind and meet my needs put me in a place of safety and balance and peace that felt like the opposite of the erotic.

So what maybe "should" have been a way in—the CARE space—was actually a dead end.

The lack of a way in was a problem I felt ashamed of. And I felt like I could never take it to my partner and get his help with it, because I didn't want him to feel criticized or in any way inadequate. When you love someone, you don't want to hurt them, both because you cherish their well-being and because, well, what if they leave you?

So I talked about it with my therapist.

She found it hard to understand at first. She—like most readers, probably, and indeed like most of her other clients—has never found that talking about science is a primary way into erotic connection. But together we boiled it down to this other really good question:

"Why does feeling loved shut you down, sexually?"

Well, I mean, hell.

My therapist knew the answer, because she had been my therapist for many years. It was so obvious, I answered with a joke:

"Are you suggesting that the household where I grew up, with a narcissistic alcoholic and an anxious, agoraphobic depressed stoic, isn't a cradle of stability and connection? Surely not!"

My therapist smiles patiently at my jokes, but she does not joke back, because she knows that under the jokes always lie the biggest, most difficult to express emotions. In this case, it was the reality that my body had learned, through the hard experience of my infancy and childhood, that love is risky and unreliable.

She said I should process all that old emotional stuff, so that I could begin to learn that *this* love is safe. I said that sounded really difficult and uncomfortable and also it would take a while and I was looking for a way into LUST *this week*, please.

She smiled patiently at that, too. She knows what the jokes are for.

Now, the "how" of therapy is both intensely dramatic and incredibly dull, because it's full of emotion and the stakes are high . . . but also it's just people sitting in a room talking about those emotions, while one of them cries a lot. So I'll summarize my process in three sentences, but imagine them with an '80s movie–style training montage, complete with motivational rock anthem:

I remembered some moments from my early life that taught me I couldn't rely on love, and I grieved for the little girl that I was, that she would never have the ideal parents every child is born deserving and no child gets. Then I talked through the ways I had grown since then, how I had honed my instincts about which people are trustworthy and which are not, about what healthy love feels like in my body, about how I was now a reliable enough "parent" to the hurt young girl who still lived inside me. I cried, sometimes with grief but also with pride at the adult I had become.

Bam. Therapy.

Meanwhile, as I did my individual work, my partner and I discovered that we had already found a new way in, one I had never shared with anyone before, one that turns out to be better—sexier, yes, but, more important, better for our relationship and better for me as a human. But I hadn't been able to see it before because I was so busy "shoulding" on myself about how CARE *should* be my way in and I *shouldn't* rely on intellectual connection.

The question we asked together was: What are we doing and how do we feel in the moments when it's easiest to say yes to sex?

The answer turned out to be laughter. PLAY. Being amused by the silliness of sex, by the seriousness most people have about it, by the entertaining nature of bodies in general and genitals in particular. They're delightful. What is laughter and joking for me? It's a room next door—or maybe it's the room right above—all the biggest, most difficult to express emotions. I could say yes to sex when both of us were willing to laugh together about the reality that I was a sexpert who struggled to drag herself off the couch and into the bed. If I took myself seriously, if I believed there was something at stake, *we were doomed,* but if I could lighten up my self-criticism and laugh at myself . . . we were freed.

And something happened over the course of our process of discovering laughter as a way in. My body began to unlearn its childhood wisdom about love as a threat. And as my body learned to trust me and this partner I was playing with, the distance between emotional connection and the erotic . . . shrank. Pretty soon, emotional connection wasn't an active turn-off anymore—that is, it didn't hit my brakes—because my brain was *unlearning* the link between love and danger.

And now?

As I wrote the paragraph about how *buh-na-naaaaaaaahhhhzzzzz* our emotional connection is . . . I turned myself on. Now I turn myself on when I write about all the ways I feel supported and accepted for exactly who I am, my oddities, my difficulties, my quirks. And, above all, for our shared sense of humor. So I ended up with *three* potential ways in! Intellect, emotional connection, and laughter—which means SEEKING, CARE, and PLAY.

(And don't forget, from chapter 2, we did the things with the door and the rug and the sex towels. Solving sex problems isn't all therapy and feelings!)

When I tried to draw my floorplan, it took me three or four drafts to find a layout that seemed to capture most (though not all) of the relationships among all my emotional spaces. Allow yourself multiple attempts. You'll learn a great deal in the process of sorting out how your rooms relate to one another.

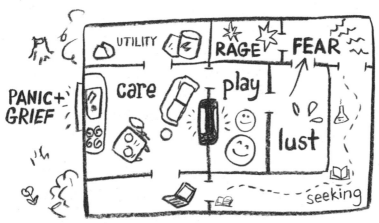

This is my floorplan. Notice that SEEKING and PLAY open directly into LUST, but I have to go through PLAY to get from CARE to LUST.

Everyone has different ways into an erotic state of mind. My sister is a musician, married to a musician, and musicians are not like other people. For them, music is in *every* emotional space in the brain—CARE and SEEKING and PLAY, but also the adverse spaces. Wherever my sister is in her emotional floorplan, there is music, and because she married a fellow musician, that means that wherever she is, she can find him. "Musicianship" is a partner characteristic that activates her accelerator, so if she's not stuck in adverse space, just listening to him practice can pull her toward LUST. The music for the audiobook of *Come Together* is a collaboration between her and her musician, and I like to think it nudged them in the direction of their room next door.

Music will never be the way in for me or my partner. We're not broken, we're just not musicians. For all I know, CARE is your room next door! People vary, and they change.

Margot and Henry

I once visited a house that had a huge indoor garden with a pool, right in the middle of the open-plan living area. It was wild. You could see the pool and garden, lit by massive skylights, from almost everywhere in the house. The entire space was pleasantly humid, bright, and bursting with greenery.

My friend Henry's floorplan is kind of like that. He constantly dwells in the vicinity of his LUST space; it's like even his pleasure-adverse spaces have waterslides leading down to this lush playspace at the center of everything.

Before I go any further with Henry and Margot's story, I want to say explicitly that polyamory can be beautiful and happy and life-affirming, as it was for Henry and Margot. And, polyamory isn't for everyone. Apart from anything else, the sheer calendar management of it all can be a big task, not to mention the time it takes to check in with everyone's feelings and make sure everyone stays clear about what's happening among and between everyone else. In a monogamous pair, at its simplest, you have to deal with Person A's feelings and Person B's feelings, plus Person A's feelings about Person B's feelings and Person B's feelings about Person A's feelings. If you add just one additional person, you also have to deal with Person C's feelings; plus Person C's feelings about Person A's feelings and C's feelings about B's feelings; A's feelings about C's feelings and B's feelings about C's feelings. But also A's feelings about B's feelings about C's feelings and A's feelings about C's feelings about B's feelings; B's feelings about A's feelings about C's feelings and B's feelings about C's feelings about A's feelings; C's feelings about A's feelings about B's feelings and C's feelings about B's feelings about A's feelings. It's not just additively complex, it is exponentially more complex. It requires time, excellent communication skills, unusually high self-awareness, and did I mention time? Trying to solve relationship difficulties by opening the relationship up to other people makes as much sense as trying to solve relationship difficulties by having a child. You might feel really good about this new person in your lives, but that doesn't mean you've actually fixed any of your problems, and now you're imposing them on someone else.

Everyone's experience is unique. But I think it's not a coincidence that the people I know who are most successful at open relationships that involve not just sexual connections but deep emotional connections are retired. They have the time, the emotional maturity, and often a couple of decades of therapy under their belts, all of which make such expansive love more practicable.

Not that Henry and Margot and their various partners over the decades never ran into problems; all relationships run into problems. In fact, two decades into their relationship, Margot was stuck in the pleasure-adverse spaces in her floorplan, while Henry was still slipping playfully down the waterslides of his emotional brain into LUST.

Margot's floorplan has LUST over in a corner, sandwiched between CARE and PLAY, with all the adverse spaces over on the other side of the house. Their "What do we want when we want sex?" answers had led them to try prying her out of those adverse spaces, pushing her toward the favorable spaces, but as we've seen so far, you get pushed into adverse spaces and have to be pulled out, just as you get pulled into favorable spaces.

"How do we get you unstuck?" Henry asked with enthu-

siastic optimism, because, did I mention, he is the Ted Lasso of polyamorous erotic connections. "What do you need?"

"Well, the first thing I need is definitely to feel like your next big project," Margot answered facetiously.

The mundane exigencies of life conspired to turn one special weekend into a slightly less special, much more convenient weekend at Margot's place. They spent the evening cooking dinner together and talking about the repairs the house needed and the addition she had been dreaming of building for a decade. At the bottom of their shared bottle of pinot noir, Margot fought sleep and lost.

"I've gotta go to bed. Can we try again tomorrow?"

"Sure!" Henry said. "I'll tidy the kitchen a little and follow you up."

He did follow her up, to find Margot already asleep. She was still asleep when he woke up the next morning.

When Margot went downstairs after ten surprisingly satisfying hours of sleep (not since perimenopause had she reliably slept through the night), she found the kitchen cleaned, breakfast warming in the oven, and Henry nowhere in sight. She took her morning dose of anti-inflammatories and then, listening carefully, she followed the muffled sound of singing and whistling to the laundry room, where she found Henry. He was naked except for Margot's flowery apron (which came to about mid-thigh on him) and pulling laundry out of the dryer, folding it, and piling it into the basket. As he folded, he danced and sang "The Wallflower," aka "Roll with Me, Henry," the Etta James Grammy Hall of Fame Award–winning hit from his childhood.

She watched him silently, not wanting to interrupt, wanting to watch his unselfconscious silliness for as long as it lasted, but eventually the dryer was empty and the basket was full, and Henry hoisted the basket onto his hip and turned toward the door.

When he saw her, he declared, "Well, good morning!"

And, well, let's fade to black on this scene, this isn't that kind of book, but suffice it to say she, uh . . . she rolled with him.

That day they learned that one path out of Margot's pleasure-adverse spaces was this delightful blend of being cared for (in the CARE space) combined with PLAY. It was the beginning of some curious exploration of unexpected strategies to get Margot out of the difficult spaces and into the pleasure-favorable ones.

Your Floorplans Are a Third Thing

Talking about your emotional floorplan with your partner is a project, a "third thing" toward which you can turn your shared attention. Doing so will not only help you create a context that allows you access to the LUST space, but it will also help to make things less stressful or fraught when either of you is struggling to get to LUST.

An example of how one couple used the floorplan: Eric, the higher-desire partner, had started to take it personally when Dana, the lower-desire partner, declined sex. Dana talked to Eric about feeling stuck in the CARE kitchen. "I'm always here! There is no path from here to sex! Instead of calling to me when you're in the sex room and I'm in the kitchen, meet me where I am and help me finish all the caregiving that has to happen in the kitchen, so I can step away! Walk with me on the path between the kitchen and the sex room, pausing in the 'office,' so I can make sure all my to-dos are crossed off and I can let go of 'taking care of' responsibilities and we can 'care for' each other!"

In this couple's case, it meant integrating householding into date night. Part of their scheduled, planned foreplay was cleaning the literal kitchen together—washing, drying, and putting away dishes, wiping down counters and appliances. I learned of this story because Dana shared with me the moment Eric, spontaneously and unasked, dried the sink with a dish towel, then put the used dish towel in the laundry and replaced it with a clean one. For Dana, this simple yet extravagant act felt exactly like being told "I love you."

Another example: A lower-desire husband's LUST space was locked up tight, doors shut and bolted, following years of scripted sex that demanded "performance" and "being the man." Both he and his higher-desire wife believed in the gendered instructions they had been taught since childhood, so they both believed his erections were a measure not only of his masculinity but also of his desire for her, his commitment to their relationship, and his ability to meet her needs in every domain of the relationship. When you shine a spotlight on a penis and demand that it perform or else, does that activate the accelerator? For a lot of people, including this guy, the pressure and performance demand hit the brakes, making erection impossible. Worse, he could barely talk about it, since even just discussing sex would be like admitting failure.

His wife learned about the emotional floorplan and brought it to him with great enthusiasm. She explained all about her floorplan, describing how each room felt for her and which rooms were adjacent to LUST. She drew it and everything, with arrows showing how she moved through one space into another.

He didn't do any of that. Explaining what it felt like to be in each room was not an option for him in that moment, he was too overwhelmed. Thinking about the relationship among all the spaces was way too much to get his head around.

But he could point at the PANIC/GRIEF space on his wife's drawing, and he could say, "I'm over here."

He was in tune enough with his internal experience to be able to identify it, even if he didn't have a lot of practice talking about it. Given a bunch of potential labels, he could match his internal experience to one of them.

His wife had assumed he was somewhere in the RAGE space, angry with her for pushing him, angry that he didn't feel in control. But when he pointed to PANIC/GRIEF, she suddenly saw that her understanding of their struggle was wrong. The solutions when a partner is in RAGE are completely different from when a partner is in PANIC/GRIEF.

Given the extremity of isolation and hopelessness that came with his experience of being trapped in PANIC/GRIEF, their next step was the right one: They went to therapy together.

"Therapy" is an answer like "mindfulness" or "compassion." Like, "*Ugh,* can't you just tell me what to do, how to fix it, instead of having to deal with all these *feelings?*"

I sure do wish I could. But great sex in a relationship that lasts decades requires your whole personhood and your partner's whole personhood. It means knowing your whole emotional floorplan and being able to talk about every room, including the uncomfortable ones. It isn't always easy. But when your partner can say to you, "I feel lonely in our relationship," even if all they do is point at a picture and say, "I'm over here," that's some powerful motivation.

One more example, because I love how varied people are. Amber (not her real name) and her nonbinary partner are nestmates in an open relationship, and she told me that both of them experience desire as mostly responsive in their shared sexual connection. But she also told me that she experiences spontaneous desire for her non-nesting partners. She said, "It's easy because, you know, I don't see them all the time and when I do it's a celebration, it's playtime, it's relaxed and fun and like recess."

Yet with her primary partner, Amber said, "We're both so responsive, it's like we're both waiting for the other one to get things started and make that, like, 'spark.'"

I said, "I'm curious what's so important about that 'spark' before other things happen."

She had a hard time explaining just what was important about the spark, so I asked a different question: "What is it that you want when you experience 'the spark'?"

Her answer: "I just want to get super-close to my partner, literally, like, smoosh up against them."

Amber's "spark" was a desire for closeness—which explains why it was easy to feel a spark for non-nesting partners whom she saw less frequently. That means her room next door to LUST is CARE—specifically, *missing* someone she cared for. If you like someone a lot and you don't spend a lot of time with them, of course you want to be closer! By contrast, it's difficult to miss someone you see every day, for many hours a day.

A pleasurable longing to be closer to someone she misses was Amber's way into her LUST space, through CARE, with a tiny dash of PANIC/GRIEF.

That made things so simple.

I said, "The usual advice is to create that spark of missing each other simply by separating from each other for a while."

She said, "Ohhh, this is that thing Esther Perel talks about. Maintaining distance."

"Right," I said. "But there are other options, too. What if, when you schedule your intimate time together, instead of thinking about it as 'How are we going to create this spark of longing?' you forget about longing and instead you try bringing all the pleasure you can to your partner? Like, 'How can I bring lots of pleasure to this person who is so amazing and great and with whom I share a huge part of my life?' That way you're not waiting for a spark, you're igniting it yourself, with CARE or PLAY or SEEKING. Stop longing to miss them, and instead long to give them pleasure."

"Oh my gosh, that sounds so much nicer!" she said.

Instead of showing up for sexytimes worried about how to create a "spark" with this person she adored, she would show up with the goal of giving pleasure to her beloved nestmate.

It was a small shift, but it was a new way in, through the room next door.

THE COST OF CONTEXT SWITCHING

I'm confident that anyone reading this is capable of making significant improvements in their sex life, regardless of how good it is already or how bad it has gotten. But I will never try to make it seem effortless, because I know that (a) lots of the things I recommend in this book take a great deal of effort and (b) knowing ahead of time that something will be effortful helps you not give up, if the going ever gets seriously tough.

That's why I need you to know about "context switching."

In both computer programming and the kind of "productivity" books that make me feel exhausted just looking at them, "context switching" is the process of switching from one task to another. This process costs time and energy. Switching to a different task or role—say from work mode to parent mode, or from parent mode to sexy mode—takes time and energy. It rarely happens spontaneously or without intention.

Our brains need to switch periodically, and different people have different needs when it comes to switching; for example, I benefit from staying in the same task for long periods of time (at the time of writing this paragraph, I've been at my desk for four hours solid), while my Attention Deficit Disorder spouse benefits from switching very frequently, as guided by his distractible but highly creative brain. He frequently has over a hundred tabs open in his web browser. For both of us, if the outside world demands that we switch our attention or maintain our attention at times when our brains aren't ready, we may be using more energy on the switch than we are on any task that we're actually working on, leaving us potentially exhausted.

Can you relate? You're in the middle of a task, finally grabbing a few minutes in a row to concentrate on one thing, and along comes a child in need? Or you're focused on a project when an email comes in or someone sticks their head into your line of sight or you get a reminder that there's a meeting in ten minutes and you need to stop your actual productive work and go be in a meeting? These are just a few of the moments when we experience the cost of context switching.

There will be times in your life when you lack the time, the energy, or both to transition out of your everyday tasks and mental states into the LUST space in your brain. That's life, that's fine.

And there will be times in your life when you have the time and energy to reach a state of whole-brain immersion in LUST, where all your attention is free to focus on the pleasurable things happening in the moment. This is the sex people want and like when they talk about freedom, when they are released into a shared spaciousness, dissolving of barriers, intense connection, and ecstasy. In my nerdy terms, what they want and like is a whole-brain context switch to the LUST room. They want to dwell there and not have to worry about anything outside that space. You probably want me to explain how to get to that state, if you don't already know. I will. That's the last chapter.

To sustain a strong long-term sexual connection, know your emotional floorplan and your partner's. Know which mental spaces are adjacent to the erotic, and know how to help each other transition out of the distant spaces, like worry and frustration, into the spaces right next door to LUST. Given all the different states of mind that have no doorway directly into LUST, it is nonsense to imagine sex should "just happen." The shift from one mental space to another takes time, effort, and energy, and we often need help from our partners to make it happen. People vary too much and the potential barriers to the LUST room are so diverse and numerous that you and your partner are the only ones who can work out how to protect that space in your relationship.

And let's never forget that sometimes you are so overwhelmed and exhausted that you can't get off the couch, then date night arrives and you just don't have enough energy left to be anything but a blob. If you're just that exhausted, here is your official permission slip not to even try to get to LUST when what you really need is ten naps and a good, messy cry. You do not owe anyone any further justification or explanation.

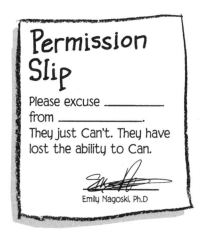

Chapter 4 tl;dr:

- Aim not for LUST itself, but for a space next door to it.

- Your emotional floorplans are helpful tools for exploring the "internal experience," part of your shared erotic context. Again, couples who sustain a strong sexual connection over the long term co-create a context that makes pleasure easier to access.

- It took me time, therapy, and the curious, supportive cooperation of my partner to help me discover new ways into the LUST space. You don't have to hurry in your exploration of your emotional floorplans.

- Moving through emotional spaces takes both time and energy. It isn't—and isn't supposed to be—effortless. It's a myth that wanting and liking sex should happen easily, instantly, and in any context.

Some Good Questions:

- Which mental states are right next door to the LUST room?

- What is my "way in" to an erotic state of mind?

- What am I doing and how do I feel in the moments when it's easy to say yes to sex?

- What am I doing and how do I feel in the moments when I can't imagine saying yes to sex?

Chapter 5

HOW WE GIVE AND RECEIVE:
A Sex-Positive Mindset

So you're mapping your emotional floorplans, learning to identify which emotional space you're in and what puts you into that space, how you get out, and where you are when you get to the other side. All of this, so that you and your partner can help each other co-create a context that makes it easy for your brains to access pleasure, especially LUST pleasure.

Let's enhance the floorplans and your context-creation with a sex-positive mindset.

For me, the term "sex positive" doesn't mean that all sex is positive (which it certainly isn't) or that everyone should like, want, and have sex. It means that *everyone gets to choose* how and when they touch and are touched, and everyone gets to decide how they feel about their body. This basic bodily autonomy is the foundation of good, great, and spectacular sex—hence sex *positive*. A sex-positive mindset acknowledges that each of us is cultivating our sexuality in a potentially toxic environment and with potentially harmful experiences in our past. Sex positivity fosters each person's sense of entitlement to basic bodily autonomy. You deserve full choice, at all times, about when and how you are touched. So does every partner with whom you share touch. You deserve to choose how you feel about your body—accepting or critical, loving or grieving—and so does every partner with whom you share touch.

Confidence and Joy

When people ask me what I do for work, I say, "I'm a sex educator; I teach people to live with confidence and joy inside their bodies."

Then they ask me if they're normal and I tell them how very normal they are.

But I wish they would ask me what I mean when I say "confidence and joy," because when you replace "Am I normal?" with "Am I confident and joyful?" your whole outlook on your sexuality shifts. Confidence and joy are the foundations of a sex-positive mindset.

"Confidence" is knowing what is true—knowing what's true about our bodies, our sexualities, our life histories, our cultures, our partners, and our partnerships. It's knowing what's true about the bodies we lust in, the world we live in, and the relationships we love in. Knowing what is true, even when it's not what we were taught should be true. Even when it's not what we wish were true.

You're reading this book to learn what's true, and this kind of education is definitely part of knowing what is true. Read books and watch videos and listen to podcasts and consume all the media you trust. But that's not the most important part of how to know what's true.

Another important part of how we learn what's true about something as complex as sex is through social learning—observing others, talking to others about their experiences and our own. You can do this on social media, but it's so much more impactful when you can do it face-to-face. There's nothing like talking to people you know and like, in real life. You learn by talking with others, as well as by reading and listening to trustworthy media sources.

But even talking with others isn't the most important way to learn what's true. The most important way to learn what's true is: Listen to yourself—your body, your heart, your mind, your soul, your internal experience. Listen, believe, and trust.

This is easier for some people than it is for others. I, for example, have a very noisy internal experience that's difficult to ignore. It draws my attention away from the external world and pulls my attention toward my own body. Yet my identical twin sister, Amelia, is *clinically bad* at listening to her body. After years of struggling with her health, she was diagnosed with alexithymia, which is basically an inability to notice or understand her own internal experience. She doesn't notice when her foot falls asleep if she sits in one position for too long. She has to think for several minutes to understand whether that sensation in her abdomen means she's hungry or she has menstrual cramps or she has digestive distress. For folks whose experiences are more similar to my sister's, she's written a "Listen to Your Body: The Basics" guide as an appendix in our *Burnout Workbook*.

So those are three ways to learn more about what is true.

But in my experience, there are three kinds of true things that are difficult to know:

1. *True things that aren't what you were taught "should" be true or things that you wish weren't true.* If you didn't grow up knowing there are brakes or that responsive desire is normal, common, and a typical characteristic of sexual connections that last decades, you might find yourself wishing you didn't have brakes, or that spontaneous desire was easy for you. It can be difficult to let go of facts that contradict your image of what an ideal sex life looks like.

Many self-help books, from home decluttering guides to professional success manuals, ask you to envision your "ideal life," as a way to establish a goal and a "why" for all the changes you're going to make. I can't do that here, because your image of an "ideal" sex life has almost certainly been shaped by a bunch of mean-spirited cultural lies. Your ideal may involve having a body or a partner that looks and acts a certain way. It may include some behaviors and not others, without reference to which behaviors bring you pleasure. It may include all kinds of "rights" and "wrongs." How many of those are something you actively chose, rather than something that was handed to you as "ideal"?

Writer and sex educator Steph Auteri wrote about her experience of learning about responsive desire and discovering the freedom that comes with knowing and loving what's true, in her book, *Dirty Word: How a Sex Writer Reclaimed Her Sexuality.*

She said to her partner, "Just because I don't want to have sex as often as you do, it doesn't mean that there's something wrong with me. . . . It's completely normal for me not to be in the mood all the time."

That was before the COVID-19 pandemic. When I talked to Steph in 2022, she told me that her revelation stuck with her for a while. She and her partner had both gotten a more concrete sense of what activated each other's accelerators and what hit each other's brakes, and things got better as they collaborated. But then, with the increased stress, exhaustion, and depression of the pandemic, her guilt reemerged. She started putting pressure on herself, even though her husband did not pressure her. That's the thing about the weeds in the garden: They can grow back if you don't keep on pulling them. And sometimes we get so busy with other things, we forget to keep weeding.

She finally talked to her husband about it, and it turned out he was genuinely okay with not having sex. The pandemic was affecting him, too. And it was such a relief to know they were both normal and his loss of desire didn't mean anything except that pandemics can make sex seem less important and less worth having.

2. *True things that other people tell you are not true.* Suppose you learn that your desire style is primarily responsive and you tell your partner, "Hey, wow, I learned this cool thing: I don't have 'low' desire; I have responsive desire!" and they reply, "No, that's wrong, desire happens out of the blue, and if you don't feel it out of the blue, then it's not desire."

They're contradicting what your own learning, your own internal experience, and your own innate wisdom are telling you is true. Best-case scenario, maybe they're doing it out of their own lack of knowledge. But also, maybe they're doing it out of a sense of entitlement to your performance of the sexual script you both thought was true for the longest time.

Let's assume a best-case scenario, where they're simply reexplaining their beliefs on the assumption that what they've always been taught is true, is actually true. This is a great opportunity to share empathy and knowledge at the same time, like, "That's what I thought, too! But I read this book by this person with a PhD and multiple bestselling books and a TED Talk and stuff, and she explained it in a way that made me understand my own experience completely differently!" You may even add, "Can I show you that part in the book?"

In an alternative scenario, where the person feels threatened by the potential withdrawal of something they feel entitled to, it's a little messier because you'll need to help them manage any sense of loss they may feel in letting go of their existing script. Some communication tips for this situation:

- Emphasize how much better your sexual connection will be when you're not trying to fight against your sexuality, you're working with it.

- Explain how much better you feel about your sexuality, now that you know your experience is normal, and reinforce that if your partner, too, can know that you're normal and not broken and thus embrace your sexuality as it is, it'll help release that judgment that was hitting the brakes, and you'll be so much freer to enjoy sex!

- Allow space for any feelings of sadness, grief, or loss that may accompany your partner's letting go of your sexuality as they believed it to be. Only by letting go of the false idea can they open up space for what's true.

3. *True things that are new since the last time you learned a lot.* This one happened to me in the form of a new medical diagnosis that no doctor or book or online advice ever mentioned might impact my sex life. I have a balance disorder that makes me so sensitive to motion that an elevator can make me motion sick. In a car, I must be the driver, I can't be the passenger. Well, while attending a plenary talk on sex and disability at a sex education conference, I suddenly realized: I must be the driver. I can't be the passenger . . . and that includes during sex. The uncontrolled motion of sex could sometimes be enough to trigger my sensitivity! But if I could adapt the way I had sex, I could avoid the triggering motion and thus avoid any potential for discomfort.

When I (joyfully!) explained my insight to my spouse, he was immediately delighted that I had figured out a way to make our connection more enjoyable.

This kind of discovery will happen over and over during a sexual connection that lasts decades. Your bodies will change, your relationship with this partner will change, your relationships with others will change, and all of these changes will create new things that are true. When you stay open to discovering new truths, you stay open to confident, joyful sex.

Some new insights about what's true can bring risk of loss and potential for discomfort, along with the joy. Coming out as gay, lesbian, bi, pan, ace, aro, kinky, poly, trans, agender, or any other of the wide variety of genders and sexualities humans experience requires you to defy much of the world's constantly expressed opinions about who you are supposed to be. Sometimes we may internalize those messages so deeply that even we can't believe anything else could be true of ourselves. And sometimes we've worked so hard to accept one identity that the idea that it could change is heartbreaking—to us, and sometimes to our partners and even to our communities because they, too, feel invested in our truth. When the truth changes or your insight changes, everyone involved needs to mourn for the truth that is now lost, so that they have space for what's true now.

Knowing what is true does not oblige anyone to share their

truths with anyone else. In an ideal world, we get to choose when, how, and with whom we explore our identities, our pleasures, and the many other domains of sexuality that may or may not be what we were told they should be or even what we once wished they were. You can be confident of what's true without being in a place—emotionally or socially—where you can comfortably live your truth out loud. That doesn't make it any less true or valid. I wish for you a place where you can share what you choose, when you choose, in a context of safety, love, and welcoming.

Confidence is *knowing what is true.*

And joy is . . . the hard part. Joy is *loving what's true*—about our bodies, our sexualities, our life histories, our cultures, our partners, and our partnerships. It's loving what's true about the bodies we lust in, the world we live in, and the relationships we love in. Loving what is true, even when it's not what we were taught should be true. Even when it's not what we wish were true.

It may seem like a contradiction, that the path to the sexuality you long for begins with loving the sexuality you have right now, as it is. If you don't love the sexuality you have right now, as it is, then you'll be so busy criticizing, judging, shaming, rejecting, and worrying about your sexuality, noticing everything you wish were different, that you won't have any time, attention, or energy left to try something new.

So here is my super-secret/not-at-all-secret-because-it-was-the-title-of-chapter-2-so-please-tell-everyone-you-know shortcut for accessing joy. When you turn away from all the various cultural lies, you can replace them with just two words of instruction:

Center. Pleasure.

Start from scratch. Assume everything you were taught about sex for the first two decades of your life is incorrect, and start again, with pleasure as your only "measure" of sexual well-being.

But let's not kid each other: Loving what's true is harder than knowing what's true, for at least three reasons:

1. *Joy is hard because we were lied to.* How can we love our orgasms if they take "too long" or require the "wrong" kind of stim-

ulation or happen less frequently than they're "supposed to"? How can we love our genitals when we've absorbed so many messages that they're the wrong size, the wrong shape, the wrong shade, the wrong smell? How can we love our sexual desire when it appears to have been missing in action for weeks or months or years or always? How can we love our bodies when our bodies are so far from what everyone in the world tells us a body is supposed to be? I hear you asking, "How, Emily, can I love what's true, when what's true is that I'm *broken* or *flawed* or *afraid* or *a failure*?"

Answer: You can love what's true because every notion that you are broken or flawed, or that your body is scary or can't heal, or that there's any such thing as sexual "failure," is a lie. You've been lied to your whole life—details on that in chapters 9 and 10, but you already know some of the lies, like the desire imperative and shame around pleasure.

It's a simple answer that I know is not always easy. When you feel yourself losing contact with joy, return to this reality: You were lied to. You *are* lovable.

2. Joy is hard because you have to "detox" from the lies. When you accept that you've been lied to, you'll feel some feelings about the fact that you've been living with lies for decades.

You may feel angry. You may feel rage at a world that deceived you for your whole life.

You may feel hurt.

You may feel sadness, grief.

None of us will ever be the person we were taught we should be. Letting go of that phantom self, we will grieve. Then the lies will tell us we are failures, that we're "giving up." And we are giving up. We're not giving up on ourselves, though. We're giving up on the lie.

These are difficult feelings.

One of the things I say pretty much anytime anyone will listen to me is "Feelings are tunnels. You have to go through the darkness to get to the light at the end."

But getting to the light isn't always easy. Joy is the hard part.

Joy is big. It's powerful. And it can be scary.

If joy is too big a step right now, especially if your body endures difficult-to-love experiences like chronic pain, loving what's true can still work if you can just reduce the degree to which you actively hate, criticize, or judge what's true. Neutral noticing is *great.* Often, neutral noticing is all you need!

Confidence and joy are the tools that make talking about sex with your partner not just easier than having sex, but potentially *fun,* because you can love what's true without judgment or shame.

Which brings me to one last thing about joy: Something I hear a lot is "*Comparison* is the thief of joy."

And that's wrong. Compare all you want. Learn more about what's true in the world, and feel free to compare your experience to other people's and go, "Ooo*ooo*oooh, that's interesting!" Comparison can be neutral noticing. Children compare their body parts out of curiosity. It's healthy and normal to want to learn more about what's true. Curious comparison is no thief; indeed, it can enhance joy.

When people say, "Comparison is the thief of joy," what they usually mean is not the comparison itself, but the judgment that can arise from a comparison. *Judgment* is the real thief of joy. When you compare and merely notice similarities and differences, you can enhance your understanding of what's true about you and the rest of the world, which increases your confidence. When you compare with positive curiosity, you can even enhance your love of what's true, which increases joy!

But when you compare not just to notice similarities and differences, but to assess and decide what is good and what is bad, who is right and who is wrong, that is the opposite of loving what is true. Judgment is deciding that some of the things that are true are bad and wrong and unworthy of equal existence. Judgment is the anti-joy, whether it's self-judgment or judging others.

"Normal"

This confidence and joy stuff might be what other people need, you might be thinking, *but, I just want to be* normal. *Not broken or a freak or a failure.*

I hear that. Literally, I hear that all the time. Some variation on "Am I normal?" is the most common question I'm asked.

But what does "normal" even mean? And why does anyone (everyone?) care whether they are normal?

I think so many people are worried about being normal because we're led to believe, falsely, that we exist on a continuum from broken to normal to perfect, like this:

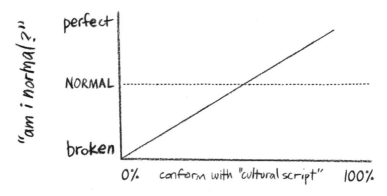

A lot of us get to adulthood believing that being "normal" is the gateway to becoming "perfect," as this graph depicts. The reality is that all of us are already normal.

We're taught that sexual "perfection" is the goal, yet no one has to ask me, "Am I perfect?" because we all already know we're not "perfect." We have decades of life experience that filled our heads with self-critical voices, constantly telling us just how imperfect we are.

So we aim for "normal," in the face of endless messages telling us we're broken, we're inadequate, we're doing it wrong, try again, no that's wrong, too, and if you don't fix it you'll never, ever be *perfect.*

There's nothing wrong with wanting to be perfect. "Perfect" is just a code word for acceptable, even admirable, and, above all, safe from anyone's contempt. Like, once you're perfect, no one can judge you.

Oh, friend. Anyone can judge you anytime, no matter how hard you work to conform to their standard.

Again, there's nothing wrong with wanting to be perfect. We all want to be free from the judgment of others. Remember, comparison isn't the thief of joy; judgment is. That includes self-judgment.

If you want to be perfect, I have good news: You are already perfect!

The linear continuum of broken → normal → perfect is a lie!

Sex is not a linear progression from broken to normal to perfect. Instead, it's a *cycle* of woundedness to healing, back to the wound, back to healing, and around again.

What wound? Maybe the idea of "woundedness" doesn't feel like your experience, but if you are trying to change your sexuality to be "normal" or to be "perfect," that longing to change, to "fix" your sexuality, is itself a wound. The wound is the lies you were taught all through your early life about bodies, sex, gender, love, and safety. It's all the self-criticism you've inflicted on yourself for not matching what you were taught you're supposed to be (much more on this in chapters 9 and 10). It's all the punishment you've survived for not matching other people's expectations. Not being "man enough" or "ladylike"; not being a strong, independent woman; not being a sensitive enough man; not having spontaneous desire; wanting sex too much; having the wrong body; not working hard enough to change your body, you slob; working too much on your body, you narcissist; being a prude; being a slut; being a virgin; having too many partners . . . However you have lived in your body as a sexual person, there have been voices screaming that you're doing it *wrong*.

With a sex-positive mindset, we turn toward what's true with love; we heal the parts of ourselves wounded by all those lies about the ways we're broken. And we turn toward what's true about our partners with love, too. With our nonjudgment and love, we help heal the parts of our partners that were wounded by all the lies about the ways they, too, are supposedly broken. In this cycle of woundedness to healing, we become stronger in the places we were hurt.

All of us have been wounded by cultural messages telling us how our sexuality "should" be, and all of us are in an ongoing cycle of healing from those wounds, then being wounded again or having an old wound reappear. Anywhere you are in the cycle, you're still normal.

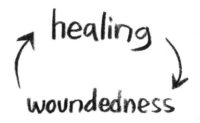

This isn't my original idea. Haven't we all heard by now that our cracks are where the light gets in? Everyone has said it in their own way, from thirteenth-century Sufi poet Rumi—"The wound is the place where the Light enters you"—to Groucho Marx—"Blessed are the cracked, for they shall let in the light." Heck, isn't the moral of every comic-book movie that our greatest strength often derives from our greatest wound?

I think when people want to be "perfect" lovers, they want to be uncracked, unwounded, not crazy. So impressively ideal that they become unleavable.

And I have not met even one person who has never been broken or wounded.

This natural, healthy oscillation from woundedness to healing allows you to transform the places you've been hurt into the places where you find your greatest strength.

The "wound" of the woundedness to healing cycle isn't just from trauma, abuse, or neglect (more on those in chapter 7), it's also all the damage done by cultural messages insisting that you're broken. They're so relentless, by their sheer persistence they actually injure or even break a sexuality that would otherwise be whole.

The very idea of "normal" has been used as a weapon against you your whole life. Even without explicitly traumatic experiences, you have been injured by the expectation of "normal."

Which . . . wait. Now we have to figure out what "normal" even means.

One definition of "normal" is something like "conforms to the expected cultural narrative."

If I ask you to describe "normal" sex, you probably have some ideas about who is having it, what behaviors they engage in, how long it lasts, how it feels, how often they do it . . . In fact, your questions about "normal" might stem from your sense that your own experience differs from this cultural script of how sex "should" be.

And let's acknowledge right now: You vary from the cultural script of how sex should be. That doesn't mean there's anything wrong with you. It's the script that's wrong. I'll say that again, just so it's clear:

Where you vary from the cultural script, it's the script that's wrong, not you.

Oh, you'd like a more scientific definition of "normal"? Okay. Here's what "normal" means in the research: If a thousand people answer a multiple choice question on a survey, the scientists add together everyone's answers to the question and divide that total by the number of people whose answers were included. That's the "measure of central tendency" or, more precisely, the "mean." In that context, "normal" would include any response within two standard deviations of the measure of central tendency.

Obviously, when you wonder if something about your sex life is "normal," you aren't wondering, "Am I within two standard deviations of the measure of central tendency?"

That's why sciencey answers to sex questions are often unsatisfying and unhelpful. For example, perhaps you wonder what the "normal" frequency of sex between couples is, in a long-term relationship, according to science? Answer: Who cares? What in the world do the people who participated in that research have to do with you and your sex life? Nothing, y'all. Bubkes. Ziparoo.

I don't answer questions like "How often does the average couple have sex?" because it's impossible to hear the answer and not judge yourself against it. If you have sex more often than "normal," you feel a certain way, and if you have sex less often, you feel a different way. It's reflexive, you can't help it. But again, what does the sexual frequency of the couples who participated in that research have to do with you, your relationship, or this season in your life? Zilchoid. Diddly-squat.

It's the same reason I don't answer the question "But how often do *you* have sex, Emily?" or "How long was your longest dry spell?" People ask these questions in search of details to help them assess their own sexual frequency or dry spell. What if I tell you we went seven years without having any sex? What if I tell you the longest dry spell was a week? You would have feelings about those two answers, because you are judging my answers against your own sex life and against the cultural script's "normal" and "aspirational" answers. As I said earlier, judgment is the thief of joy.

So when people ask me any version of the question "Am I normal?" the answer is yes.

Oh, you're pretty sure there are exceptions and you want a precise definition? Okay!

"Normal" sex is any erotic contact among peers, during which (a) everyone involved is glad to be there and free to leave whenever they choose, with no unwanted consequences, and (b) no one experiences unwanted pain.

"Glad to be there" doesn't have to mean "I can't wait!" It can be as simple as "Hey, buddy, nice to see you." "Free to leave with no unwanted consequences" means not just no physical consequences but no *emotional* consequences. No guilt or shaming, no emotional bribery ("but if you loved me you would . . ."), no coercion of any kind, not even "Aw, c'mon!" If your partner pouts and complains if you want to stop doing something, that might be commonplace, but it's not part of my definition of normal sex.

If you're the partner who's glad to be there and your partner wants to change or stop what you're doing together, you may experience uncomfortable feelings like disappointment, frustration, or fear of rejection. Those feelings are normal, and when your partner is ready you can talk about them. But isn't it so much better to feel some frustration and worry, rather than find out your partner wasn't glad to be there and was only going along with it because they didn't want to hurt your feelings? Hurt feelings are so much easier to cope with, so much easier to heal, than the hurt of having sex when one of you is not glad to be there.

And "no unwanted pain." If you're experiencing pain you enjoy, do you, friend! Whether you're being spanked, whipped, clipped with clothespins, pierced, stretched, or having your hair pulled, if you enjoy it in a context of mutual consent, go for it. But if it hurts and you dislike it, that sensation doesn't belong in normal sex. There are any number of medical conditions that can cause pain with sex, and your best course of action is to find a great medical provider. I say this knowing that it often takes multiple tries (especially for women, especially for women of color and women with disabilities) to find a doc who will take our pain seriously.[1]

But "unwanted pain" includes unwanted emotional pain, too. If your eroticism includes the experience of being, say, humiliated, scolded, punished, or ignored, and you and your partner are participating with mutual consent in that experience, *awesome*. As the kids say, I'm loving that journey for you. But if you feel humiliated, scolded, punished, or ignored by someone you're connecting with erotically and you didn't choose that dynamic together, that's not part of my definition of normal.

So. When you find yourself worried if you're normal, now you have a way to tell.

But just as people aren't asking if they're within two standard deviations of the central tendency when they ask me, "Am I normal?" they also aren't asking me, "Is my sex fully consensual and free of unwanted pain?"

So what *are* people asking when they ask, "Am I normal?" "Is this normal?" or "Is my partner normal?" And why does it seem to matter so much? After all, you're not reading a sex book in order to be a "normal" lover, right? If your partner told you after lovemaking, "That was really normal sex," would you feel complimented?

In my experience, when people ask if they're normal, they mean, "Am I broken?" "Am I doing it wrong?" "Am I adequate?"

"Do I belong within the human community, or am I a freak and a failure?"

Without knowing anything about you, I can already answer those questions: No, No, Yes, and You absolutely belong within the human community.

None of these questions can be answered by learning about other people's sex lives and then judging yourself in comparison to them. As I say again and again, everywhere I go, we are all made of the same parts, just organized in different ways. And all of those ways are beautiful, normal, and—dare I say—*perfect.*

Abandon the idea of "normal" as the gateway to "perfect." Normal, by its usual definitions, is a dead end. Replace it with the cycle. Here in the real world of woundedness to healing, "perfect" *is the cycle itself.* Anywhere you are in the process, you're in perfection.

You're not satisfied with that. That's fine. You want a definition for "perfect" sex? As in, "the best" sex? Okay, I'll give you a definition:

The best sex, *perfect* sex, happens when everyone involved is not only glad to be there and free to leave with no unwanted consequences (i.e., normal sex), but also when everyone involved turns toward their own and everyone else's sexuality, as it is right now, in the moment, with confidence, joy, and calm, warm curiosity. (Curiosity is the subject of chapter 7.)

For example: Suppose a partner with a penis wants an erection and isn't getting an erection. Both of you turn toward that soft penis (and toward all the feelings you each have about it) with confidence, joy, and calm, warm curiosity, loving what is true. You enjoy the pleasurable experiences you can have with a soft penis, whether that means playing with the soft penis or directing your shared attention elsewhere. That's perfect sex, regardless of whether or not an erection happens!

Another example: Suppose you want to have an orgasm and you've been stimulating yourself off and on for something over an hour and you haven't gotten there, despite high levels of pleasure and arousal. Turn toward that pleasure and arousal with confidence and joy. Love what's true. Perfect sex, regardless of whether orgasm happens!

Perfection lies not in solving every problem, permanently; that will never happen. Because it's a cycle, you will always be moving through woundedness and back to healing and back to woundedness, growing with each cycle, even as life circumstances change and affect how you grow and heal. Perfection means you are always growing, always healing, always changing, always confronting new ways to grow.

Mike and Kendra

Mike's recognition of the woundedness to healing cycle started out as a conversation in the kitchen while Kendra got dinner ready.

The kids were with their grandparents and due home any minute, but obviously Mike and Kendra seized the opportunity to have a ~~fight~~ conversation. But as they began to cover the same ground they had covered at least fifty times before, Kendra's patience wore thin.

He wanted her to want sex, she was sorry but it wasn't that easy. Mike didn't resent that exactly, buuuuut . . . well, haha, if he couldn't have passion, he would take what he could get, he told Kendra for the fifty-first time, with a heavy sigh and eye roll.

(Allow me to draw some foreshadowing attention to the heavy sigh and eye roll. It will turn out to be the key to the whole thing.)

His exact words were "I'd rather have sex when you're not super into it than not have any sex at all." Spoken like "Hahaha aren't men absurd with how much sex matters to us? Aren't we silly?" He was making fun of himself, making light of his unfulfilled, four-year longing.

But that's when Kendra lost patience. She turned away from her grated carrots, raised her voice, and said, "Are you seriously telling me that you would rather have sex with me when I'm not into it than have no sex at all?"

Nonplussed by her strong reaction, Mike said, "Why? It's not—"

"And how many women before me did you have sex with when they weren't really into it?"

She was glaring at him with a mix of rage and disgust.

Mike was silent. His face was cold and his hands were shaking. At last he said, "You know that's not what I meant."

"No, I don't. I think that's exactly what you meant, because it's the words you said. 'I'd rather have sex when you're not super into it than not have any sex at all.' That's what you said." She turned away from him, back to her cutting board. She grated carrots for the salad.

"I was joking, I was trying to lighten the mood."

"Look how well that worked!" she shouted as she grated. "The mood is so light right now!"

"Why is this such a big deal for you?" he said.

She dropped her knife and turned back to him.

"Are you listening to what you're saying? Are you hearing yourself? You're telling me you can enjoy sex with someone who's just going through the motions. You're telling me that it's worth your time and energy to have sex with somebody who's writing a grocery list in her head the whole time? Really? You like that?"

"I don't like it, I just . . . shit." Mike stood with his hands on his hips and turned his face to the ceiling, to keep back tears. "Shit."

"What?" Kendra snapped.

"I hear what you're saying, but—"

"Oh, 'but.' But what?"

"But . . . I would never actually like sex if you weren't fully agreeing. What I was feeling is . . . I just need to feel I'm accepted, I'm acceptable. And sometimes . . . with you, yeah, I'll take what I can get and be grateful."

On other days, Kendra might have melted into compassion and tried to make him feel better, assure him that he is accepted and acceptable. Right now, though, she was in no mood to coddle his feelings. She said, "You can't get that from any of the other things we do together?"

"I can, but sex is like . . . it's ultraconcentrated acceptance. It's a big dose of 'you're not disgusting or ridiculous, actually.'"

See that? The real feeling underlying Mike's longing was to feel like his sexual desires, his sexual body, were lovable, rather than contemptible.

Relenting just a little, Kendra acknowledged, "And here's me saying that your haha-super-funny joke about having sex with someone who isn't super-stoked to be there is—"

"Both disgusting and ridiculous. Yeah," he said. He sniffed and opened the fridge door to browse for a snack.

"Eat a carrot if you're hungry; dinner's almost ready," Kendra told Mike, then added, "Sorry. You're not one of the kids. Eat whatever you want."

They were silent for a few minutes, as Mike ate a slice of carrot, allowing the tension to dissipate a bit, before Kendra said, "Is there really no midpoint between me treating you like sex with you is gross and me treating you like sex with you is the thing I want more than anything in the world?"

"I—"

They heard her mom's car pull into the driveway, signaling the return of the kids.

And they let it go for the time being.

These kinds of conversations are complicated and have lots of layers—how everyone feels right now, how everyone feels about the history of the situation, how everyone feels about the various potential solutions—and you may be thinking, "All they need to do is X" or "Why can't they see that Y?" They can't see what you or I see, because they're in it.

But some things were already going really well with their communication. What most impresses me about Mike in this conversation is that he got to the vulnerable, hurt part of himself without Kendra having to act like his therapist or his mother. She didn't have to be sweet and help him along; he felt the painful source of his longing, even when she was frustrated. He didn't yet know what to do with it, but he recognized at last that his desire for Kendra's desire was not about her, it was about a deep, old wound inflicted on his sexuality by a culture that doesn't teach men how to receive love.

Mike wanted passion. He wanted spark. But under that, he wanted to be received by his long-term sex partner as not repulsive. He would have to heal that wound before he could fully let go of his wish for Kendra's spontaneous desire, and he would have to let go of that in order to open himself up to the project of co-creating a context that prioritized pleasure over any specific experience of desire.

I know some readers will be feeling joyful, free, and delighted by this alternative way of thinking about their sexuality—not as a standard you're supposed to try to meet, but as a personal exploration with no good or bad, no right or wrong, apart from consent and no unwanted pain. But others may be feeling frustrated, disappointed, dissatisfied, or annoyed. You want concrete, practical strategies for solving problems that are damaging one of the most important relationships in your life, and here I am talking about confidence and joy. Maybe it sounds frivolous.

But in fact, this is the most concrete and practical advice I've given so far in this book. The others are just information. This one is transformation. Unlearn the lie of linear progression from broken → normal → perfect and replace it with the woundedness to healing cycle. Change what the words "normal" and "perfect" mean to you. The research and my own personal experience, as well as the reports from many, many students, all agree that loving what's true and flowing through the cycle is how you build a great sexual connection that lasts across many years.

The elements of a sex-positive mindset require an ongoing challenge to old patterns that no longer serve us. If what you've been wanting is to match some idea you have about what sex is "supposed" to be, what you really need is to be who you truly are. Don't aim for change right now. Aim to know and love what's true right now. Pleasure will grow from that.

I know it's not necessarily intuitive. If you don't believe me, that's fine; try it anyway. Try it for six months, collaborate with a partner, give it your all, and if it doesn't improve your sex life, email me and tell me all about it.

In the meantime, we'll end with some great questions to ask yourself and your partner.

Chapter 5 tl;dr:

- Confidence and joy are essential components of a sex-positive mindset. Confidence is *knowing what's true* about your body, sexuality, relationship, life history, and culture. Joy is the hard part; it's *loving what's true* about your body, sexuality, relationship, life history, and culture. Even if it's not what you were taught "should" be true. Even if it's not what you wish were true.

- Many of us grow up believing that sex exists on a linear progression from broken → normal → perfect. It doesn't. Instead, sex exists within a cycle of woundedness to healing, and none of us is ever "finished," we are all always moving through the cycle.

- "Normal" sex is any erotic contact among peers where everyone involved is glad to be there and free to leave with zero unwanted consequences, including emotional consequences, and where no one experiences unwanted pain, either physical or emotional.

- "Perfect" sex is normal sex where everyone turns toward whatever is happening with confidence (knowing what's true), joy (loving what's true), and calm, warm curiosity.

Some Good Questions:

- What was I taught "normal" sex is? Who has it, what do they do, how often, where, and why?

- What was I taught were the consequences of failing to be sexually normal?

- In what ways is my sexuality not what I was taught it should be?

- How is my sexuality like my partner's? How is it different? Which differences are easy to notice neutrally, and which differences activate a sense of judgment—that one of us is wrong or right, broken or normal?

Chapter 6

WHAT WE GIVE AND RECEIVE:

Trust and Admiration

Sometimes, sex with a long-term partner happens spontaneously, but most of it happens on purpose, which means that most sex will require that you *communicate* about plans, obstacles, and pleasures with your partner.

Fortunately, you already communicate about all kinds of practical things with your partner. You may communicate about work hours, meals, chores, kids, coordinating time with other partners, other friends, other family. And those conversations aren't always easy and unemotional; people have feelings about work hours, meals, chores, kids, and time with other people. If you can have those conversations, you can learn to have sex conversations. But if communicating about sex were the same as communicating about all those other potentially heavy topics, I would not need to devote a third of this book to it.

Because of the damage done to us by cultural lies (on these, much more in chapters 9 and 10), many of us feel like it's easier to *have* sex with someone than it is to *talk* about it with them.

This chapter will help you get to the "having sex" part more easily, by explaining the relationship characteristics that make it easier to talk about sex.

Whether a relationship is sexually exclusive or not, regardless of the genders of the people involved, there are some basic, necessary dynamics that make it easier for each person to participate in cultivating a shared garden. In this chapter, I'll talk about two relationship characteristics that are crucial.

They are: admiration and trust.

Admiration

What are some of your favorite things about your partner? When do you most enjoy their company? What makes you proud to be their partner?

In chapter 2, I suggested we all only ever have sex we like. Here, I want to suggest that we all only ever have sex with people we like.

Sound obvious? Stay with me.

A therapist at a workshop asked me what I would suggest for a couple that was choosing to stay together "for the kids," though they didn't like each other. They agreed that they didn't like each other. Yet they still wanted to have sex.

I was baffled at first. I asked, "Why . . . sorry, why would they want to have sex with someone they don't like?"

"Well, that's a good question," the therapist answered, and she wasn't being facetious. She had been working with the couple's assumption that the husband in particular deserved sex, but if he was still married "for the kids," then his wife, whom he disliked, was his only source of sex, so they needed to find a way to have acceptable sex with someone they disliked.

I offered the only advice that seemed ethical to me: If spouses dislike each other to the point of just waiting until the kids are out of the house before they split up, they're also waiting to have sex they'll enjoy until the kids are out of the house. If those partners show up at their shared erotic garden and they both think, *Ugh, this asshole again,* when they see their partner . . . I understand that they might manage to have some kind of sex, but how can they have sex that's actually worth the time and effort?

The world would be a better place if we all only ever had sex with people we *like.*

Being able to look at your partner and see them as admirable, even when you may be in a difficult emotional space like RAGE or FEAR or PANIC/GRIEF, is essential to co-creating a satisfying long-term sexual relationship.

In a way, what I'm suggesting here is extremely basic and obvious, right? You have to like each other most of the time.

But also, it's a radical shift in priorities. I'm replacing "passion" and "spontaneous desire" and "being in love" with the seemingly tepid emotion of "admiration." It takes me back to the myth that RAGE and LUST can co-exist in a functional long-term sexual connection; we have been taught that somehow intensity matters more than valence—that is, the sheer quantity of emotion is more important than whether that emotion feels good or bad.

Certainly there are people who have experienced and even aspire to feeling "passionately in love" with their partner, without regard to whether they admire that person.

Whenever you find yourself prioritizing passion over admiration, remember the most common thing people want and like when they have sex is *connection.* You can have sex with someone you don't admire, of course you can. But if you want to sustain a multidecade sexual connection with someone . . . why connect over and over with someone you don't admire? Won't you just feel more and more alone, as you reinforce the lack of emotional engagement between you?

Admiration is a great benchmark for choosing a partner in the first place, and for those who share a household with a partner, admiration is a great tool for getting through the inevitable rough patches. When we are stressed, our brains are more prone to noticing the things that annoy or frustrate us and ignoring things that please or impress us. If you're exhausted and irritable and your partner brings you flowers, your brain might think, *Sure, like flowers are going to help the situation,* whereas when you're rested and calm and your partner brings you flowers, your brain is more likely to think, *Flowers! My partner thought about me when I wasn't with them, and they went out of their way to bring me a gift!*

When you are stressed, remember that you chose this person—maybe even to the exclusion of all other sex partners. Surely there was a reason for that. Admiration is an important component of a sexual relationship that you would like to last decades, because, honestly, why bother talking to each other about your emotional floorplans, or about what you want and like when you want and like sex, or about your brakes and accelerator, if you don't admire the person with whom you're collaborating to create that shared sexual connection?

If you sometimes, or often, can't find much to admire about your partner, don't despair. You are not alone. It's so easy to forget to admire our partners, in the midst of the hullabaloo and frenetic planning, scheduling, and "Can you please just run the laundry?!" of daily life. And there are evidence-based ways to strengthen your sense of admiration in your relationship. Here are two:

The first is an exercise I learned when I dragged my spouse to a Hold Me Tight weekend workshop (based on Sue Johnson's Emotionally Focused Therapy [EFT]—10 out of 10, by the way, highly recommend). It was John Gottman's "I Appreciate . . ." Adjective Checklist. It's a literal list of positive adjectives, and our job was to select a few that were "even slightly" characteristic of our partner, "even if there was only one instance of this characteristic."

Notice how gently this language prods couples in the direction of noticing the good stuff, since partners might be doing this exercise while they're in the midst of a lot of conflict.

When you consider your partner, maybe the first thing you'll think of is all the things you resent, all the complaints you have. Set that aside for a few minutes, and instead consider some characteristics about your partner that you appreciate.

Here's a second exercise that can help: Think of something

about your partner that drives you up the wall. (The first time you try this, choose something that drives you up a very small wall; leave the "makes me question my life choices" problems for when you've got more practice.) Then consider what trait underlies that behavior and think of a way that same trait shows up positively in your relationship.

For example, I joke with my partner that I am perfect—my perfection lies in my "imperfections." What I mean is: All the best things about me are inextricably tied to the worst things about me. (By "worst," of course I mean all the things I'm most inclined to beat myself up for.) Do I forget important dates, ignore household tasks, and fail to express gratitude to him for picking up all the slack I leave? I do. Do I also have intensely focused attention that lets me do stuff like write books, stay finely attuned to him when we're in an erotic place, and learn new things to make our lives better? I do. And all of those things are tied together. I wouldn't trade my intense focus for anything . . . but I also feel bad when I forget important tasks.

The same goes for him. Some of his best traits—his loyalty and kindness and reliability and humor and sensitivity—are inextricably tied to the ways he sometimes struggles. He's the clutterbug in the family, because he's loyal to any object that enters the house. He'll do anything I ask, because he is kind, but I can't just say, "Hey, I need this thing"; he benefits when I pad my request in tenderness and light, because he is sensitive. The emotional labor he requires of me feels entirely worth it because his sensitivity is one of my favorite things about him.

Try reframing a partner's imperfections, flaws, or shortcomings in terms of a link to that partner's greatest attributes:

Stubborn → Persistent

Unfocused → Free-thinking, creative

Demanding → Believing we deserve the best, together

All the best, closest-to-perfection traits about you are linked to the most difficult traits about you, too.

Exercises like these develop what therapist Sara Nasserzadeh calls "emergent love," love that emerges through shared experience.[1]

They are why I fall more "in love" (whatever the heck that even is) with my person every year. As we struggle together through whatever vicissitudes life offers, we learn each other's strengths and needs better and better; we support each other according to our own strengths and we acknowledge our needs more and more fluidly.

I've offered two ways to enhance mutual admiration in your relationship. But let's spend a moment addressing a challenge therapist and author Terrence Real calls "normal marital hatred."[2] It happens when a trait that may have been charmingly quirky at the start of the relationship becomes intensely irritating. It's often the result of having to live with the charming quirk day after day, month after month, year after year. Maybe you roll your eyes at the way your partner makes the bed. Maybe you can't take the way they channel surf or let a show run continuously on streaming even when they're not watching anymore. Admiration is an inoculation against the irritation, so you can avoid the escalation of these mundane irritations into full-blown hate; it gives you practice at remembering the good things about your partner, even when you're confronted with the not-so-good things.

For example, I interrupt my spouse. Like, a lot. At least once a day. I feel like I know his mind so well that I know what he's going to say, so I skip ahead to my answer before he gets his thought out. It's very irritating of me. Fortunately, he knows that my rudeness is a product of the same traits he finds admirable in me, like my quickness of mind and my sense of deep connection with his thought process.

Without the admiration, it might be easy to assign some other meaning to the quirk. He could decide I'm doing it to annoy him. He could wonder if I'm deliberately disrespecting him or don't have enough patience with him even to let him finish a sentence. He could turn it into a power struggle. But in reality, it's just a less-than-thrilling part of what it means to share a home with me, a person he admires, trusts, and loves so much.

Other tools beyond admiration can help, too. Hatred lives in the RAGE space of your emotional floorplan, so you can process the flash of RAGE when you know how you move yourself out of the RAGE space. In fact, my simple definition of "hatred" is that it's RAGE motivation to destroy something that is in your way, standing between you and some goal you're moving toward. Like the goal of finishing a sentence. Now, people have a lot of feelings about the word "hate"; there are a lot of "shoulds" around it, which makes the phrase "normal marital hatred" seem really flashy—we're not supposed to hate people, especially not people we love. Feel free to replace "hate" in your mind with "frustration" or "irritation" or "annoyance," but all of those emotions live in the RAGE space, which means a tool you already have that can help you is simply knowing how you move yourself through the RAGE space into a different space.

But if the interrupting (or the sexual difficulty) becomes a character in a larger story about respect or power or trust, it feeds our sense that the interrupting (or sexual difficulty) is symbolic of some relationship-threatening problem. Just as interruptions cannot, on their own, end a long-term committed relationship, sexual difficulties can't either. It's when we wield the interruption (or sex problem) as proof that there is something fundamentally intolerable about our partner that we begin to spiral away from normal hatred or irritation into a darker place.

Even in my relationship with—confident hair flip—genuinely superb communication, we can't always reach each other. But there's something we always do right: We can laugh at us.

For example, here's another way that I am *so* irritating: The highly focused attention that helps me write big books also means that sometimes when my beloved spouse talks to me, I do not hear him. And when I do hear him, I can pay attention for a couple of minutes before my attention is tugged back to whatever I was focused on and I've tuned him out again. Do I *try* to keep my attention on him when he needs it? I absolutely do! But sometimes my brain just can't disengage from what I'm doing. People vary.

He has developed playful strategies for managing me. Sometimes he counts how many times he says what he wants to say before I notice he's there, and then he says it again. "Have you been there long?" I'll ask, if he seems to be suppressing giggles.

Or sometimes he'll begin the conversation with total nonsense until I notice that he's talking. "Have you ever thought about how delicious pizza would be if cheese was on the bottom?" is a real example of something he has said that I did not hear. He told me about it when I asked him for an example just now.

And that's my third trick. The first was to recall how the quirk is related to the things you admire about your person. The second is to remember how you move through the RAGE space. And third, when you're outside of RAGE, go to PLAY.

Just as it would be easy to assign meaning to frequent interruption, it would be so easy for him to take my highly focused attention personally. It would be so easy for him to start telling himself a story that it's *impossible* that I genuinely do not hear him, I must be ignoring him on purpose, I'm being rude, disrespectful! Instead, he thinks it's hilarious. How can a person so smart and responsive be so truly oblivious?

Intense experiences of anger are rarely funny in the moment, but often, after the fact, if we can stop taking ourselves so seriously, it can be hilarious. If you're thinking, *But it's not funny, it's serious!* then it's not just normal marital hatred, it's a conflict about something outside the scope of a book about sex in a long-term relationship.

We love our people for all the things they are and all the things they aren't. We celebrate the things they are, and we laugh over the things they aren't.

Ama and Di

Ama and Di might seem like an odd fit, on the surface. Ama is Black, from a pretty affluent family, spiritual, and approaching her fortieth birthday. Di is nearly fifty, white, raised in poverty, secular, and autistic. They met online fifteen years ago, on a message board discussing the works of Octavia Butler.

Di was diagnosed with autism—ASD Level 1—in her late thirties, when Ama, then an anonymous internet-message-board friend, suggested she might be on the spectrum. Perhaps a giveaway: It did not occur to Di to be offended by the suggestion. She just scheduled the appointments, got the diagnosis, and then spent a solid year re-evaluating the meaning of everything that had ever happened in her life.

Di drives Ama bonkers sometimes, in ways they attribute to Di's neurodivergence. For example, anytime inflation makes her grocery budget unviable, Di goes through a period of mentioning how much each item used to cost when she was a kid.

"A box of mac and cheese costs a quarter," she said, as her wife picked up the organic kind with extra fiber and pasta shaped like animals, even though it cost six times as much as the store-brand kind right next to it.

Ama and Di both had good incomes. They could afford what Ama called "food food." Di knew this; she didn't mention the prices because she was worried about money, she said these things because it's part of her brain's process of rewriting her inner understanding of the food budget.

"A can of tuna costs like a quarter," she mentioned as she scanned unit prices and Ama picked up the line-caught solid white tuna in oil.

"We're paying for more than full bellies," Ama replied unnecessarily. "It's also the environment and the nutritional value and—"

"I know, honey. I agree with our choices," she said. And later, "Eggs were seventy cents a dozen."

"From battery farms with inhumane conditions, sold in those Styrofoam containers that will exist until the end of time!"

"I know. I agree this is better. . . . Ground beef was a dollar a pound."

Normal marital hatred.

Di had never experienced it and didn't understand it when Ama brought it up.

"You hate me?" Di asked, bewildered.

"No, I would never use the word 'hate' to describe what it feels like. I just have a little rush of annoyance or frustration each time you talk about food prices, but sometimes it floods, like when there's been a lot of rain but everything is fine until one day it's not and suddenly the basement is underwater?"

Di nodded, trying to understand. "You want me to stop talking about grocery prices when I redo the budget?"

"Yes, that would be nice," Ama said. "But really I want you to understand what it feels like to me when you do it."

Di nodded some more, but said, "What does it feel like?"

"It feels—and remember, I know that this is not your intention, I know you're just in your brain, clicking away, but it feels like you're shaming us for not prioritizing frugality over other variables when we make food choices. It feels like you're flashing your childhood poverty in my face, instead of simply appreciating that we are in a position to prioritize environmental variables and nutritional variables and even just flavor preferences over how much something costs."

"All that, from me just saying historical prices?"

"Yeah. All that."

"It's a lot."

"And again, I know it's not your intention. It's just how it lands for me."

"Heard, love. Should I try to just write it down instead of saying it out loud?"

"That would be great."

This is one simple strategy for addressing the small things that can generate big feelings. Ama explained what the small behavior felt like, the meaning that her own internal experience imposed on Di's words. She felt understood by Di, and Di recognized the importance of shifting this small be-

havior. She looked for simple ways to make space for what Ama needed.

Sometimes she did need to say it out loud, though, but she found she could say it to her older kids, who rolled their eyes but hey, they learned a little about Mom and a lot about inflation and wage stagnation in the face of growing income inequality.

The key takeaway here is that they have the same dynamic when it comes to talking about sexuality. Remember their conversation in the shower, when Ama told Di she realized that what she liked was playfulness and teasing? And Di did that and it worked? When you can ask for what you need in a way that's clear to the person receiving the request, problems get solved without resentment or defensiveness. And that sure is a lot easier if you admire your partner, instead of believing the stories your mind creates about why a person might be doing something that drives you bonkers.

Trust

The most evidence-based couples therapies put *trust* at the center of their programs, for good reason. Trust is so much the foundation of any connection that the absence of trust is essentially the absence of connection.

So what the heck is trust, how do you build it, and how do you repair it when there's a betrayal?

Researcher and therapist Sue Johnson breaks trust down to the question "A.R.E. you there for me?" A.R.E. stands for emotionally *Accessible*, emotionally *Responsive*, and emotionally *Engaged*. Notice that trust is *emotional*, not intellectual. It's not a rational decision, it's an emotional dynamic between and among people. It's about being there for your partner, not just physically, but with your heart.

When you're asking yourself about the trust in your relationship, powerful questions to begin with are, "Am I there for my partner?" and "Is my partner there for me?" Are you emotionally present for each other?

Underlying this dynamic of being emotionally *there*—accessible, responsive, and engaged—for our partners is our *willingness to bear some cost* in order to benefit our partners or our relationships. In the examples I'll share here, that cost comes mostly in the form of making considerate choices about your communication and allowing moments of difficult emotions—yours or theirs—to be a normal part of a long-term relationship.

EMOTIONAL ACCESSIBILITY. Sometimes trust is damaged by a specific crisis event, like a betrayal. But more often, emotional accessibility erodes gradually, through neglect, as partners grow emotionally distant. There are plenty of good reasons why a couple might experience this. The sheer overwhelming demands on our attention from our jobs, our kids, our families, the world in general, may leave little for our partners. Or we may feel so stuck in the adverse emotional spaces of PANIC/GRIEF, FEAR, or RAGE that we can't find a way to transition into emotional presence with our partner. Just as we have to choose to engage erotically with our partner, cordoning off space, time, and energy for it, we have to choose to engage emotionally.

Trust-eroding overwhelm and stuckness were important ingredients in my own sexual dry spell. My attention was drawn away from my relationship to my work, and as a result I wasn't there for my partner. He agreed that my work was important and he was able to meet his own needs, and he didn't want to "burden" me. And I didn't want to burden him. By the time I had the wherewithal to reengage, he had gotten into the habit of doing everything for himself, not connecting with me, not collaborating. Not "burdening" me. So had I. And if each of us could meet our own needs autonomously, why would we open back up to trusting each other, relying on each other to be there? Why try sharing the emotional weight we were each carrying, when we knew we could each get by independently?

The answer to "why" was, well, we got married because we agreed that the other person would be our main person for the rest of our lives. Though we were still each other's main person, we were disconnected by each person's autonomy. It wasn't that we didn't trust each other, it was that neither of us was willing to take the risk of asking our partner to bear a cost for us. We could just co-exist in the same house, without asking each other to do the emotional work of being emotionally accessible, which is what differentiates our connection with each other from our connections with anybody else.

Our solution was not about repairing trust but *rebuilding* trust, remembering to ask our partner to be emotionally accessible to us, despite the fact that it was actually more effortful, at first, than just coping independently.

If you and your partner are "roommates" rather than partners or lovers, you may have grown into this habit of independently coping and not relying on each other to be emotionally accessible. A good place to start in rebuilding emotional accessibility is John Gottman's "stress-reducing conversation" technique, where you and your partner spend half an hour every day, fifteen minutes each, listening to each other's experiences, especially complaints about other people. The listening partner listens not to solve problems but to be a cheerleader, to be on the same team as the speaker. Be there for each other emotionally. Practice not coping independently but daring to cope interdependently.

EMOTIONAL RESPONSIVENESS. When partners are struggling with responsiveness, a common culprit is plain old distraction. Our attention is tuned to a screen or to the kids or to other friends or partners or family or to work or to any of the myriad things we have to pay attention to. Because of the cost, in effort and time, of context switching, we offer our partner a fragment of our attention as we continue to think about something else.

But when nonresponsiveness accumulates over time, it can escalate into a spiral of resentment.

For example, some straight friends of mine, let's call them Jeff and Susan, were trapped in a dynamic of rapidly escalating conflict. In just a few sentences, they could transition from Susan calmly asking Jeff to clean the kitchen, to enraged yelling.

How did they get there? By failing to be responsive to each other's emotions.

Jeff was not emotionally responsive to Susan. Instead of responding to her requests for help, he would ignore her until her requests became so irritating that he responded just so she would be quiet. Thus Susan learned, over many years of his lack of emotional responsiveness, that the only way to get his attention was with huge, intense emotion. It wasn't just the kitchen, of course, it was many things. Above all, it was *what it meant* that he cleaned the kitchen, what such an act of householding symbolized about his sense of investment in their relationship. And she had to yell in order to see him invest even the smallest amount of time and energy.

The same dynamic played out in their sex life, with the roles swapped. Susan, resentful and disengaged, would ignore Jeff's bids for sex until his requests grew so persistent, critical, and annoying that she would agree to sex, just to make him stop asking.

How would you feel if a partner agreed to have sex with you just to shut you up? Wouldn't it be more satisfying if they were enthusiastic rather than resigned?

This situation is often treated as comedy, the nagging wife and the lazy husband. The "frigid" wife and the horny, entitled husband. But in reality, there's nothing funny about it.

A loved one's lack of emotional responsiveness is basically a form of torture for humans. In the renowned Still Face Experiment, originally conducted in 1975, mothers were coached not to respond to their infant's interactions and bids for attention.[3] No eye contact, a neutral facial expression, no touch. After just three minutes without response from their parent, with repeated attempts to create the usual reciprocal back-and-forth of parent-infant interactions, the babies grow wary, withdrawn, and sad. They go into PANIC/GRIEF, experiencing a tiny wound to their CARE space, and also, crucially, experience the hopelessness that comes with losing a sense of self-efficacy.[4]

Self-efficacy is an individual's sense that they can engage with the world in a way that results in getting their needs met. A simple and familiar example of self-efficacy is knowing you can get a snack from a vending machine. A bag of candy getting stuck in the machine is a reliable source of outrage because the unfairness of it challenges our sense of self-efficacy. Like the "nagging wife, lazy husband" trope, this situation is often treated as comedy, and fair enough. The stakes are low. It's just a bag of candy.

But in a sense, the candy isn't just candy any more than cleaning the kitchen is just cleaning the kitchen. The trapped candy is a symbol of our self-efficacy, our sense that we know how to engage with the world so that our needs are met. So we laugh in recognition, at the idea of someone escalating to rage, helplessly attacking an unresponsive machine. But Jeff and Susan were escalating to rage and helplessly attacking their unresponsive spouse.

Yet their relationship withstood their spiraling failure of emotional responsiveness. How? Therapy, yay! They had spent years with nonresponsiveness eroding the trust between them; at first, they didn't trust each other enough to believe that the other would truly show up for the project of rebuilding trust and neither was willing to take the risk of trying, when, it seemed, the other person was unwilling to take the risk of trying. It took the support of a professional to help them grieve the old hurts and practice being there for each other.

John Gottman describes this "nasty-nasty" state, where both partners are in an adverse emotional space, as the place "where the couple's love and fun go to die."[5] In this state, he defines trust as each partner reliably changing their own behavior, even if it costs them something to do it, in order to make it easier for the other person to transition out of their negative emotional space.[6] For example, Jeff learned that when they were stressed and annoyed and bickering, Susan would crack a little joke at her own expense, so they could laugh a little—a transition toward PLAY. And she learned that Jeff could pause, take a deep breath, and give her a hug—a transition toward CARE. He might add some PLAY, saying, "Imagine if we had to get through this with some other loser instead of each other! Ugh!" Even if they both still had unresolved difficulties, they would each do a little emotional work, bear a little cost in order to make it easier for the other person to transition into a better state.

EMOTIONAL ENGAGEMENT. When partners are emotionally engaged, they turn toward each other's feelings with a warm "yes." Just as failures of responsiveness are often about distraction, common failures of emotional engagement are about *communication skills,* like advice-giving instead of active listening, or "I'm busy" instead of "I'm here for you." That's good news, because it means it's not a failure of trust or trustworthiness itself; it's just a matter of practicing the skill of listening to your partner's feelings.

When your partner comes to you with a difficult feeling and you offer advice for how to solve the problem that caused it, you're engaging with the problem instead of engaging with your partner and their feelings. And you're allowed to do that, but you're missing an opportunity to enhance emotional engagement and thus develop mutual trust. When you approach your partner to initiate sex and they say a reflexive "no" because they're busy or not in the mood or they're still resentful from some disagreement you had earlier, they're engaging with the question of having sex right now (even if you're trying to initiate for later tonight or later this week) rather than engaging with your feelings about having sex. They're allowed to do that, but they're missing an opportunity to enhance emotional engagement and thus develop mutual trust.

I struggled with this for a long time. I understood the principle of emotional engagement, but it just seemed so *inefficient* to spend a bunch of time talking about our feelings! Can't we just solve the problem and move on? Can we just say yes or no, without having to talk about *why* yes or no, or how both of us feel about the yes or no?

Then I learned a deeper layer to listening to feelings, a layer that gets less attention. I share it here for everyone who, like me, wants communication to be efficient.

Individual differences in temperament is most often studied in children and babies as young as newborns, but it remains pretty stable across a person's whole life.[7] A variety of temperamental traits can affect how intuitively we respond to our partners with emotional engagement, rather than with problem-solving, criticism, or "no." I'm going to describe just one: *adaptability*.

The temperamental trait of adaptability is about how readily we adjust to changes and transitions. Some people transition readily from task to task, from setting to setting, from role to role. But maybe you've spent your whole life feeling really stressed when you transition from one task to another, no matter how familiar those tasks are, or from one setting to another, or from one role to another, so when your partner presents you with a potential transition—for example, if they invite you to have sex—something inside you grinds with resistance, just because of the difficulty of transitioning out of whatever state of mind you're currently in, into a sexy state of mind. Remember the cost of context switching I mentioned at the end of chapter 3? That cost is higher for you, if you're slow to adapt.

If you're slow to adapt, your first response to a partner, say, initiating sex, isn't necessarily a no or a yes, but a sigh or a groan at the effort you know it will cost you to stop watching this television show and start moving toward the LUST room, even though in the past you've almost always been really glad you made that effort.

People who take more time to adapt prefer to have a plan, feel comfortable with routines, and like to know what's going to happen ahead of time. They might be people to whom the idea of scheduled sex is naturally appealing. "Yes, let's put it in the calendar!" What they might not recognize is that they don't need to schedule just the sex, they need to schedule the *transition* into sex. Shifting from work mode or parent mode or hobby mode to LUST mode takes time and energy, as you learned in chapter 3 with your emotional floorplan. Your necessary skill is:

Learn what helps you transition.

What do you do to disengage from one mode to another, from one task to another? You have successfully done it in a variety of areas in your life, so you know you can do it in this area, too.

Maybe you use music to transition, or a bath, or a change of clothes. Maybe it's being playful about your struggles with transitions; maybe you flop dramatically on the sofa and say, "I can't, a dragon came by just now—it was pretty amazing, I'm sorry you missed it, but it cast a spell and turned me into this blob of jelly, you have to roll me off the couch and into the bedroom."

Partners of people who are slow to adapt can know not to take it personally. Some people just adapt more slowly than others and benefit from more structure around transitions. In a partnership where one person makes transitions much more gradually than the other, emotional engagement happens when the faster partner expresses support, instead of impatience or judgment, during the transition. In a sense, the faster-to-adapt partner bears the small cost of patience and adapting to their partner's needs, while the slower-to-adapt partner bears the small cost of learning and practicing smoother transitions. Emotional engagement is making a plan and helping the slower-to-adapt partner know what to expect, through the creation and protection of a routine. And the beautiful, ironic reality is that the more trust a slow-to-adapt person has in a shared routine, the freer they'll feel to be flexible.

If your partner needs more time to adapt than you do, a little advice: There is no speeding them up. Trying to hurry them along will only slow them down. But if you instead adopt the mindset that planning and preparing for sex is part of the fun, like planning a vacation is part of the vacation—an opportunity to daydream about what it will feel like when you get there—then it will be easier for you to enjoy the transition process and frame it as part of the sexy play you share, instead of a chore to get over with before you finally get to the sex part. Trust your partner to transition at their own pace and they'll trust you in return.

For some of us, trust is easy because we learned it early, in our families of origin. For others of us, trust is so, so hard. If trust or being trustworthy are difficult for you, you know what I'm going to suggest, right? Therapy. Therapy and books.[8] This stuff is deep and sometimes difficult, but if we're willing to strengthen our psychological foundations, we build a more stable platform from which to launch our erotic explorations.

Chapter 6 tl;dr:

- You don't need to want your partner passionately so much as you need to like them, admire them, and believe they are worth some effort on your part.

- Trust is essential to a strong relationship, and it is not rational, it is being *emotionally* there for your partner—being emotionally accessible, emotionally responsive, and emotionally engaged. As researcher and therapist Sue Johnson puts it, "A.R.E. you there for me?"

- Communicating with trust and trustworthiness isn't always efficient, but it is always more effective. Take the time to be emotionally present, especially for difficult feelings, and you'll improve the foundational strength of the relationship.

Some Good Questions:

- What is easy to admire about my partner? About myself?

- What might be difficult to admire about my partner, but is inextricably linked to one of their most admirable qualities?

- If I bring a difficult feeling to my partner, what would their ideal response look like?

- If my partner brings a difficult feeling to me, what would my ideal response look like?

- Am I there for my partner, emotionally accessible, responsive, and engaged? Is my partner there for me? When trust feels weakened, what do we do to repair it?

PART 2

Good Things Come

Chapter 7

LIVING IN BODIES

Sometimes it's easy to dive into erotic connection because the context has already made it easy to access pleasure—when our relationship is thriving, when we're relaxed and happy and healthy. Other times—when we're stressed or ill or raising small children or in a big fight about money—the context makes it difficult to access pleasure. Couples who sustain a strong sexual connection over the long term treat their shared context as a shared project, with the goal of making it easy to experience pleasure.

Here in part 2, I want to help you manage the barriers you're likely to face as you put this into practice in your own relationships. If "pleasure is the measure" was the moral of the story of part 1, the moral here is:

Good things come.

. . . To those who wait, I mean.

Co-creating a pleasure-favorable context isn't something we do in a day. Our sexuality is a garden; it has seasons. There are times when our most life-affirming choice is to harvest the fruits of our erotic connection, yes. Other days, deep in winter, the life-affirming choice is browsing seed catalogues to prepare for spring, which always comes, whether we're here for it or not. Just like pleasure, we can always cultivate change; we can never force it.

We are not promised abundant time, in this life. But we are promised *change*. The key to sustaining a strong sexual connection over the long term is to adapt—with confidence, joy, and calm, warm curiosity—to the changes brought by each season of our lives. Even in the face of the difficulties we'll confront in this part of the book, you and a partner can co-create a context that makes pleasure not just easier to access, but abundant and ecstatic.

In this chapter, our focus is on the ways that difficult aspects of living in a body—illness, pain, disability, aging, and so on—can actually enhance an erotic connection!

Let me qualify that.

One time I met a militant vegan who told me that actually? vegans have *more* food choices? because they can eat *all these plants*.

To which I replied, "But omnivores can eat all those things, and also meat and eggs and cheese . . ."

To which he replied something rude that I forget, but basically he got mad.

I say this to illustrate that I am not someone who frames limitations as Better, Actually™. Just because you experience a major health issue or trauma doesn't mean you automatically have access to special sex magic that you didn't have access to before.

But let me revisit that conversation with the militant vegan and offer the best faith interpretation I can of his words:

It's not that vegans have "more choices," it's that the limitations set by their diet create a context that encourages them to explore, try new things, and embrace experiences they might have passed by before.

And that's true for an erotic connection with a person whose illness, trauma, or aging changes their needs. You may not have "more choices," but you do have a context that encourages you to explore.

Try new things. Shed all the preconceived ideas about how sex "should" work and experiment with all the ways it can and does work for you and your partners, in the bodies you have right now.

In this chapter, we'll apply this idea to three potentially difficult aspects of living in bodies: the changes we experience in our health status, the shame we carry from early life experiences, the trauma many of us did not choose but were forced to experience.

Calm, Warm Curiosity

The fundamental mistake people make when they approach change is that they approach the problem from a RAGE space, trying to destroy it; or they approach it from the FEAR space, trying to solve it by pretending it doesn't exist; or they approach it from PANIC/ GRIEF. When you're in PANIC/GRIEF, you desperately need to ensure your continued existence by repairing a relationship, or else you're lost in the darkness of helpless isolation. Trying to solve a sex problem from a PANIC/GRIEF space is how people begin having sex they don't necessarily want or like, for the sake of salvaging a relationship.

Ultimately, the reason problem-solving from an adverse space is ineffective is that RAGE or FEAR or PANIC/GRIEF are *reactive.* The problem activates a stress response that motivates you to destroy or run or spiral, rather than to explore, understand, and feel compassion.

SEEKING, by contrast, is *creative.* In her book, *You Belong,* mindfulness teacher Sebene Selassie noticed that "reactive" and "creative" are the same word with the C moved.

"What does the C stand for?" a friend asked her.

Curiosity, was her answer.

She writes, "Curiosity is a crucial component of lessening our reactivity. Rather than react out of habit, we become interested. But how do you cultivate curiosity if you get pulled into reactions before you even know it? How can you be curious about your unconscious conditioning? How do we meet any moment with creativity instead of reactivity? Easy—we stay open to our experience. Okay, it's not that easy. But it's possible."

It's possible, with practice. In the language of the floorplan, staying open to our experiences is witnessing our own internal experience from OBSERVATIONAL DISTANCE.

In fact, curiosity is an important tool for giving us just enough distance from our RAGE, FEAR, or PANIC/GRIEF, to be able to find our way *out* of those spaces.

Here is your way out:

"I see you. I love you. I want to know you."

Hello, problem. Hello, struggle. Hello, wound.

Calm, warm curiosity is a blend of three spaces on your emotional floorplan: SEEKING, for curiosity, CARE, for emotional warmth, and OBSERVATIONAL DISTANCE, for calmness.

We begin from OBSERVATIONAL DISTANCE. "I see you." When we approach a problem, our first step is to shift into our scenic viewpoint, to see the situation as if we're viewing it from the outside. When we create distance between ourselves and the problem, we can be neutral, nonjudgmental of ourselves and our partner.

Then CARE: "I love you." This is our turning toward, with an urge to care for, rather than correct or corral, a problem. CARE is a loving space from which to seek solutions. Does it seem strange, to love something you want to change? Think about it this way: If a child is crying, does yelling at them to stop crying help? No. You turn toward them with love, to soothe the distress. It's the same when you turn toward your own struggle.

And finally SEEKING: "I want to know you." Moving toward, exploring, "Ooh, neat! what's that?"

What might happen if you approached your body and your partner's with calm, warm curiosity? Let's find out.

Bodies Vary and Change

If you're lucky enough to grow old with a partner, you'll have the glorious privilege of watching them age and granting them the privilege of watching you age. To be in a long-term relationship is to be with someone as they go through times of wellness and times of disability. Stay with someone long enough and you may well find yourself in the role of caregiver as well as lover.

Lots of people have these kinds of experiences, at every age. We live in bodies; bodies are liable to damage and are inextricably tied to illness and mortality. I have friends who had cancer in their twenties and relied on their partners, in relationships much shorter than mine, to help them through the side effects of radiation, surgery, and chemotherapy. My sister's husband has been through a dozen surgeries, and she herself has been hospitalized multiple times and, most recently, was a COVID long-hauler, experiencing chronic fatigue and pain for years after she was technically "recovered" from the infection. They have had to be there for each other in basic, biological ways for a large proportion of their two decades together.

Maybe the big diagnosis comes into the relationship with you— your partner comes into your life with a disability, chronic illness or pain, or you come to your partner with something.

A curious approach to illness or disability will help you to see the illness or disability as something separate from your partner. Your partner *has* needs, but they are not their needs. Stay present with your partner; see them, not just their needs.

Shane and Hannah Burcaw are an interabled couple with a YouTube channel chronicling their experiences. Shane was born with spinal muscular atrophy; he uses a wheelchair and needs assistance with tasks of daily living. Hannah watched a documentary about him, felt they had a lot in common, and emailed him out of the blue. Shane says of that email, "She used parentheses in a way that did it for me."

They often address other people's ableist assumptions about their intimate life. These comments derive from people's apparent inability to recognize that you can be a caregiver and a lover within the same relationship. It's not a sacrifice; it's not "noble." It's what you do when you love someone and share a life with them for years. The couple has a sense of humor about it—in a series of question-

and-answer videos, they used the word "intimacy" as a blanket term to cover all sexual behaviors, so they don't have to go into specific, awkward detail, but Shane invents names for fictional sex positions, like "flaming flamingo" and "Alabama snakerider."[1]

In addition to the funny parts, the pair offers deep wisdom any relationship can benefit from. When asked how they "draw a line between affectionate touch and caregiving touch," they answer simply, "We don't draw a line. There is no line. Not even imaginary. We just go back and forth between the two." Shane adds, "We don't say, 'Okay, caregiving is over, and let's begin the intimate touch. Caregiving will involve intimacy. Sometimes it will, sometimes it won't. Intimacy will involve caregiving here and there, like 'Hannah, can you move my leg to the left?' It's all intertwined and the same."

Hannah offers this analogy: "You can give your significant other a high five and that's not a different relationship than when you're being intimate."

In an interview, they described their sexual connection as the kind of sex life I would wish for any couple.[2]

"Our intimacy benefits from my disability," Shane says. "It doesn't look like what you see in the movies, maybe, but like I can totally do it."

Hannah says, "In general Shane just uses his voice in ways that other people might just physically do something."

"I will just say, 'Hey do you wanna go have sex?'" Shane agrees. "And I know that that probably strikes people as like, 'Oh, that must be, like, not romantic, but like, take our word for it. After I ask that, we're romantic. When we're in bed together, I can say like, 'Hey, can you roll me towards you or can you move my arm so I can reach your neck or cheek?'"

Hannah continues, "And we have shorthand for all these things. Like you're not just saying, 'Can you please put your legs up under my legs?' I feel like I just know his body and preferences as well as I know my own."

And there's my whole book that took me years to write, laid out in a couple of paragraphs: It doesn't look like in the movies, but we talk to each other about what we want and we know each other's bodies as well as we know our own.

Got that? That's pretty much what you need to know.

Jessica Kellgren-Fozard and her wife, Claudia, are another inter-abled couple and a delightful example of caring for without falling into the trap of "taking care of." Jessica has two genetic disorders, one affecting her nerves and another affecting her connective tissue, together causing an array of differences and health issues, including deafness, chronic pain, migraines, chronic fatigue, and occasionally accidentally dislocating a joint or completely losing mobility in her limbs. Claudia does not have any genetic health conditions—though she is very grumpy before her morning cup of tea. Like Shane and Hannah, the couple married in their twenties, and physical challenges and accessibility were a part of their relationship from the very beginning.

In a two-part video, Jessica and Claudia address the assumptions strangers make about their relationship, particularly ableist comments like "Your wife must be an angel, you're so lucky to have her," and "Your conditions must be so exhausting for your wife," as if Jessica were a burden for a loved one to carry, rather than a person and a partner who contributes to a relationship.[3] No, the couple clarifies, Jessica is quite a catch, actually, and they both contribute the best of themselves to the relationship.

They answer questions like "If Claudia is sick or hurt or something, does she ever feel like she can't complain about it because you are still worse off?"

Before Jessica has even read the whole question, Claudia is already side-eyeing the camera and shaking her head. She answers, "No. That's a firmly resounding no," and Jessica cackles and adds, "No no no no no no no." In fact, they say, Jessica really loves looking after people and Claudia really loves being looked after, regardless of the actual physical needs in the relationship.

Jessica is Jessica, who loves to bake and dance, regardless of her current physical situation. And Claudia is Claudia, who loves to garden and travel, regardless of her current physical situation.

While they make the entirely valid choice not to be explicit about their sex life in public—boundaries for the win!—there is nothing about the way each of them looks at the other that disguises their adoration, admiration, and tenderness. They see each other, and they don't let the needs called for in a specific situation obstruct their loving gaze.

Wait, isn't this a sex book? Why is this big section about pain, injury, disability, and illness in here?

Friend, this is a book about sex in long-term relationships. If you're not already in an interabled relationship, if you stay with someone long enough, eventually you will be. I know a lot of us are used to advice about how to "spice things up," but we know from the research that adding stimulation to the accelerator is only occasionally what's needed to keep a sexual connection engaged. More often, we need to eliminate the things that are hitting the brakes. And some of the things that might hit our brakes are out of our control, so instead of changing the thing that hits the brakes, we change how we *feel* about the thing that hits the brakes, so that it doesn't hit the brakes anymore.

Speaking of changes over the long term: menopause. If someone in your relationship has a uterus, menopause will probably happen at some point, whether medically induced, surgically induced, or biologically induced. While there's no specific uterus-related hormonal situation that influences your sexuality directly, lots of the changes that come with perimenopause and menopause can impact sexual functioning. Hot flashes, unpredictable menstrual cycles, changes in how your body stores fat, the fact of aging itself, gender dysphoria, all of these might hit the brakes. A stray comment from a partner about the changes to your body can activate an overwhelming cascade of feelings about yourself and about your need for support from your partner. Beyond that, reductions in estrogen can alter the lining of the vagina, making the tissue fragile, which can increase pain with both internal and external genital stimulation, which in turn can reduce sexual desire, since, again, it's difficult to want sex that hurts. Vaginal suppository medication can help with the tissue issue, but that has to be supplemented with gentleness and patience, unlearning the link between genitals and pain. Fortunately, as Gen X ages into menopause, we are rejecting medicalized and gendered ideas of what menopause means and how to experience it. Heather Corinna's book *What Fresh Hell Is This,* and Omisade Burney-Scott's multimedia *Black Girl's Guide to Surviving Menopause,* are part of this shift, integrating intersectional, trans- and nonbinary-inclusive social justice lenses to the endocrinology, psychology, and social experiences of menopause.

Our own changing body and our partners' don't have to hit the brakes, unless we decide to hold on tight to cultural assumptions that say bodily changes and needs disqualify us from being sexual.

A writer friend of mine, who was a nurse for many years, says, "Illness creates the deepest intimacy." Giving and receiving care is the essence of our human need for connection. "Caring for" gathers a loved one into a supportive embrace. "Caring for" holds the loved one in one hand and their needs in another. "Taking care of" risks losing sight of our partner and noticing only their needs.

Illness creates the deepest intimacy. What that intimacy does to your erotic connection depends on whether you can still see your partner as your partner through their illness, and whether your partner can still see you through yours.

Margot and Henry

Margot and Henry were experiencing normal aging: menopause, less rigorous erections, body changes like Margot's rheumatoid arthritis and coronary artery disease for Henry, not to mention life stressors that belong exclusively to the lucky people who live long enough to experience them. Margot was a grandparent, Henry a great-grandparent, and some of their own kids and their kids' kids and their kids' kids' kids had struggles that Margot and Henry wanted to be there for.

Between the physical challenges and the emotional stressors, it was no wonder Margot was feeling stuck in CARE, unable to relax into PLAY or SEEKING.

Margot harnessed some advice she remembered from a

grandchild's school counselor, to figure out what could help her and Henry co-create a context that made it easier to access pleasure.

"Four kinds of social support," Margot reviewed, "Instrumental, Informational, Emotional, Appraisal."

(Ultra-short summary for those who don't spend much time with school counselors or public health employees: Instrumental support is giving concrete aid. For example, if you're hungry, I give you a Fruit Roll-Up. Informational support is imparting knowledge or teaching a skill. Example: You're hungry, I tell you where to find the Fruit Roll-Ups or maybe I teach you how to make them. Emotional support is being there, emotionally, for someone, in all the ways we described in the Trust section. For example, if you're hungry and there's no immediate aid available, I am there for you, with empathy and compassion, helping you sustain hope until a concrete solution is available. Appraisal support is offering feedback about a person or their situation, in order to help them change that situation. For example, you tell me you're hungry and I, as your therapist or your best friend, suggest some characteristics in your personality or life history that are preventing you from accessing the food that would otherwise be available to you.)

"So," Margot said, "what are some things we already know make it easier to get to the sexy?"

"Emotional support!" Henry crowed. (Ted Lasso of polyamory.)

Margot added, "Actual instrumental support. Helping me get done allllll the different tasks and chores and errands. The more we can get off my plate, the easier I can walk away from my day."

"That's amazing, isn't it?" Henry said, surprised. "It didn't occur to me that the cleaning and things weren't just symbolic, they were real things that were really weighing on you, and if I just do them . . . it's almost like your sexual brakes have a to-do list, and if we just check some things off,

your brakes are freed up enough to let the accelerator fly free!"

"Yes. That's news to you? Okay. Thumbs-up for informational support."

"I guess I was thinking it's the thought that counts."

"It's not that the thought doesn't count, but a basket full of folded laundry and an empty kitchen sink actually eliminates *things that were hitting my brakes, rather than just being nice about the things that were hitting my brakes."*

"What if we pretend I'm the plumber come to fix your leaky faucet, and you slide your fingers down my crack?" Henry batted his eyelashes at her.

Margot laughed but said, "There's another level to it, too. Dishes and laundry and fixing the leaky faucet are things I used to be able to do easily on my own. But lately . . ." She stopped and rubbed at her knuckle joints, a familiar gesture to both of them. "The pain hits my brakes, but, more than that, it reminds me that my body is not what it used to be. I worry that I'm losing my independence. And when you can do those things for me, without my even having to ask? That's emotional support and instrumental support all in one. It releases me from the difficult emotions and makes it easier for me to get to pleasure."

Understanding different ways to create a supportive connection was part of their process of co-creating a context where pleasure was easy, as their bodies changed. But I do want to add that they worked on the erotic context itself. Much as my husband and I put sex towels near the bed, Margot and Henry bought some supportive pillows to make various positions easier, including positions that made giving oral sex easier for both of them. They also used tools like cock rings and strokers (short, soft, often silicone tubes that enclose the shaft of a penis) to make hand jobs less of a strain. And they followed the one and only prescriptive advice I give: Use lube. Not the usual drugstore kinds, the fancy-pants "body safe" lubes you get at specialty stores or online.

Since they weren't worried about using latex, Margot and Henry chose coconut oil as the most comfortable on her menopausal genitals.

It's not all big feelings and conversations. Sometimes it's lubricant and pillows and pocket pussies.

The Dark Places Created by Shame

A lot of us have fraught relationships with pleasure. Over the course of our lives, we're likely to be shamed or judged for some parts of our sexualities. In response, we hide those parts, even from ourselves. They live in what I call the "dark places," shadowy corners of yourself that you don't even want to look at. The woman in chapter 3, who was groped and then was triggered by her partner? Her brain's response to the trauma was to build a trapdoor that opened into FEAR, a dark place, whenever it recognized a sensation similar to the unsafe experience.

But dark places can also come from unremembered shadows cast on our infant bodies.

A woman told me this story that illustrates the origin of a dark place in one person's body: She had read *Come as You Are* and was thinking about its messages about body image and shame, when she watched her brother changing his baby daughter's diaper. When the baby was clean, he reached for a fresh diaper, and when he turned back, she was touching her genitals.

He scolded her, "Ah-ah! Don't touch that!"

How might he have responded if his baby had a penis instead? Would he have scolded his child for touching those genitals?

How might he have responded if his baby had been touching her feet, instead? Don't we love it when babies find their feet and play with them, as they explore and get to know this new body they were given?

This baby will not remember this moment, but it will accumulate with countless similar moments to create a dark place in her mind. She will associate her genitals and their sensations with the

experience of being scolded or punished. Her genitals make her a
"bad girl." By adolescence, she'll have a sense that that part of her
body does not truly belong to her, that the sensations of those
parts are dangerous or disgusting. Maybe her entire LUST room will
be dark, windowless, airless, full of unopened suitcases and dusty
skeletons. And she may not even remember any explicit message
from anyone, telling her to feel ashamed.

Dark places make themselves difficult to find by design. Some
may be disguised, so that your mind just glides past them without
noticing. Some may be guarded by armed and angry monsters,
so that your only response is to run away without even trying to
explore.

Sex educator Nadine Thornhill was already an expert in child
and adolescent sex education when her three-year-old son, playing
in his room with a friend, was discovered by the friend's mom; the
boys were showing each other their penises.

The friend's mom told Nadine what happened and was very
calm about it, knowing, as Nadine knew, that this kind of thing was
just a normal part of being a kid.

And yet.

As Nadine told me, "I was so ashamed and had this visceral
angry reaction and I yelled at my son, but then later I was like,
'What did I just do to my kid?'"

She soon realized, "Ohhhhhh, I just totally got triggered and
became the mean mom who yells at her three-year-old because
that's what happened to me."

What happened to her?

When she was five, she was at a babysitter's house with the babysitter's two sons, who were about her age or a little older. They
were playing in the basement when one of them said, "Let's all pull
down our pants and look at each other."

Young Nadine said, "I don't want to," but the boy tried to talk
her into it and eventually said, "I'll go first." He pulled down his
pants . . . and that's when his mom walked in.

The mom asked her son, "Why are you doing that?"

And the boy said, "Nadine wanted to do it!"

"Did you, Nadine?"

Little Nadine shook her head vehemently, but the other brother chimed in, "Yeah, Nadine wanted to do it!"

So five-year-old Nadine got dragged upstairs and sat on the couch and lectured about how wrong and bad and dirty she was. She was going to a birthday party later that day, so she was dressed up in her pretty birthday party dress. She sat in her birthday party clothes, crying, and received the shaming excoriation as she thought, *I would never say that, because I'm all dressed up!*

When she got home, her mom asked what had happened, and thankfully Mom believed her side of the story.

Yet, Nadine told me, "There had been a tiny part of me that was curious and wondered what would have happened if I had done it. And that stayed with me for years, like for *years.* I would feel ashamed if I just felt curious about sex. If I inserted myself into a fantasy, my brain would be like *nope,* so I had to insert some kind of avatar for myself in the fantasy."

But the shame's interference with her fantasies was not a catalyst for turning toward that ancient shame with curiosity so she could unpack it, discard it. It was only when she saw herself yelling at her young child, just as she was yelled at, that she saw the importance of being curious about it.

It was a revelatory, transformational moment, but not in the way you might think; her whole life wasn't suddenly changed as she instantaneously shed the old hurt. It wasn't the moment when everything changed . . . but it was the moment she decided to change everything.

She was already working as a child and adolescent sex educator, so you'd think if anyone had the tools and resources to deal with this on her own, it would be Nadine, but no. What she did have was knowledge about how to get the support she needed to do the work that had to be done. So, as many of these stories end, she said to herself, "I need to get into therapy. I've heard about 'breaking cycles,' but I don't know how to do that, so I'm going to find a professional."

Parenting can trigger old shame and pain, and she didn't want to behave toward her kid in ways that were shaped by hurtful experiences she never chose for herself. That was what motivated her to turn toward her dark places with curiosity.

When you come upon a dark place inside yourself, you may have feelings about it before you even begin to explore. You may feel a sense of dread or foreboding, a sense of anxiety and a desire to run or hide, or maybe the hot flare of anger that tells you something dangerous is there.

If that's your experience, don't try to "push through" those uncomfortable feelings. Those uncomfortable feelings are part of the dark place. Rather than push through, *breathe* through. Stay with the difficult feeling. Turn your attention toward those difficult feelings with . . . you guessed it: calm, warm curiosity.

Confidence is knowing what is true, and that includes knowing the difficult truth that we live in a world where sex may be used as a weapon against a person and where anyone who doesn't fit the prescribed "norm" is shamed and punished for their sexuality.

PS: No one fits the prescribed norm. We have all been shamed and punished. That's why we *all* have dark places—and it's also why some folks are unaware of their dark places. We hide them even from ourselves . . . and then when something goes wrong in our sexuality, we have no idea why, because everything we can see about our sexuality looks fine.

The dark places may be among the most difficult things to know about ourselves and to love. And don't worry about "finishing" the process of shining a light on all your dark places; you may never get there. You don't have to. Turn toward your dark places with warm curiosity; it will grow easier each time.

Trauma, Neglect, and Abuse (Oh My)

As a sex educator, I have some pretty wild fantasies, but maybe not the kind you think. For example, I have a fantasy that one day I'll write a book about sex and not need to include a section on trauma. I'll be able to dwell in all the pleasurable, optimistic, joyful delights available to us through our sexualities.

As it is, at least one in three of the women, one in six of the men, and half the trans and nonbinary folks reading this likely have experienced some form of intimate partner or sexual trauma. Trauma isn't limited to a response to an isolated incident, like a specific attack. It can also emerge in response to ongoing abuse, where someone feels trapped in a relationship (sexual or not). Beyond sexuality itself, *neglect* can do as much damage as a specific violent incident. Childhood neglect is slippery because it's so easy to tell ourselves stories about how it wasn't neglect, it was autonomy, our adult caregivers needed to work that much, they were struggling themselves, etc., etc. All of that can be true, while it's simultaneously true that your little body didn't get its needs, including its need for CARE, met enough to prevent emotional injuries. About a third of people experienced sufficient childhood adversity, including neglect, to significantly impact their health and relationships as adults.

That adds up to a large proportion of the population walking around with deep wounds, chronic emotional pain, and related physical health consequences.

So here we all are. Hi, everybody, hello. Me, too. Welcome to the biggest party no one wants to be invited to.

But it *is* a party. We're over here shedding the experiences that taught us we didn't deserve to be safe. We're out in the garden, folding rich, fertile compost into the barren places where someone hurt us. We're celebrating survival, grieving and raging and rediscovering ourselves, together. In literal terms, we're going to therapy, reading books about healing, cultivating loving, trustworthy connections, practicing self-compassion or, when that's too difficult, compassion for others and for our younger selves.

Your experience of trauma, neglect, and/or abuse (TNA, for short) probably influenced your emotional floorplan. I don't know what your brain did to survive, but here are a few of the patterns you might notice—though, again, everyone's brain is different and reacts in a unique way to TNA.

Your CARE space might have a randomly appearing space-time portal into PANIC/GRIEF, so that anytime you're in CARE, you could blink and suddenly find yourself in PANIC/GRIEF. Or your CARE space might have a poorly constructed floorboard that breaks when you step on it and you find yourself plunging into either RAGE or FEAR. You'll notice that in the floorplan of my emotions, there's a one-way door from LUST to FEAR. This is how my brain coped with my own trauma.

Recall the diversity of experiences included in that FEAR space. It's not just running away. It's not even just cowering in a corner, trembling until the threat goes away. It can also be people-pleasing, perfectionism, and a need to keep everyone around you happy at all times, regardless of the cost to yourself. That's a stress response sometimes known as "fawn," and it can be a trauma response, too. FEAR can also be "freeze," a dull, numb, checked-out feeling. I've seen this one appear in people's eyes while I talk to them. They come up to ask a question about a difficult experience they had, I begin to answer in a gentle but frank way, and it's like they depart their own eyeballs. They look like they're listening, but their TNA has grabbed their rational brain, said, "Nope," and hauled them off into PANIC/GRIEF or a freeze FEAR response.

The ways our brains adapted to TNA are not ways we are broken; they are ways we are survivors. Our emotional floorplans got us through. Maybe some of those TNA adaptations aren't as helpful these days; maybe we'd prefer to make some changes, now that we're not in immediate danger. We get to choose.

There are whole books about sex and survivorship, and if your TNA is affecting your sexuality, I hope you'll explore some of them, and maybe pursue therapy.[4] But here, I want to offer a specific tip for survivors, which is that sometimes our "escapist" behaviors are actually part of our healing:

Be curious about the metaphors and stories that soothe you.

Nothing in our real lives can explain or describe what happens inside us as we heal from trauma. We may *need* the metaphors of a fantasy world to describe our experience.

Take *The Lord of the Rings*. A thousand pages of high fantasy, plus two volumes of mythopoeic stories. People don't reread all that because it's fun to spend that much time with a bunch of white men of different statures. People reread it and memorize ancestries

and learn to speak fictional languages because they need somewhere to be that feels the way they feel on the inside; and nowhere
real feels like what trauma feels like on the inside.

Frodo the hobbit says, "I will take the Ring to Mordor.
Though . . . I do not know the way." That can be what it feels like
to choose to heal from trauma. Every morning when we wake up,
we decide to carry this burden another step closer to wherever it
can be destroyed, even though we don't know where we're going
or how or if we'll get there.

Why do people love Samwise Gamgee? Because though he can't
carry the Ring, he can carry Frodo. He is an ideal co-survivor: he
stays, no matter how scary it gets; he suffers alongside Frodo, but
he never equates his struggle to his friend's. You want to know how
to help a friend with their trauma—or feel what it would be like to
have an ideal supporter? Check out Sam, who wants to go home to
his Rosie, but he would never abandon Frodo.

The best metaphor for my own TNA is *Moana*—a Disney car-
toon musical, which I, a fortysomething woman, saw three times in
the theater. When something grabs you so hard you have to see it
or read it or listen to it many times, be curious about what that
metaphor is doing for you.

Moana is called by the ocean to cross the horizon and restore
the Heart of Te Fiti—a green stone that was stolen from the goddess of life and abundance. For me, the big moment is when Moana
confronts her last, worst enemy, the lava monster Te Kā. When I
see Te Kā rise up in fury, my brain goes, *It. Me.* I'm watching my
best self, as Moana, approach the most difficult and damaged parts
of me, as Te Kā. And what does Moana do? She notices the swirl
on the chest of Te Kā, a swirl that matches the swirl on the Heart
of Te Fiti. She sees below the surface of Te Kā's rage, and instead of
being afraid, she turns toward her. She sings, "They have stolen the
heart from inside you / but this does not define you. / This is not
who you are." She puts the Heart of Te Fiti at the center of the
swirl on Te Kā's chest; they touch foreheads, breathe each other's
air, and . . . the lava monster transforms into Te Fiti, the goddess of
life and abundance.

And I stare at the screen, eyes wide, tears dripping down my face into my snack. Why?

Because this metaphor explains, more accurately than any literal description can, what healing feels like for me. Like Moana, I see beneath the surface of my own pain; I turn toward it without fear, with calm, warm goddamn curiosity. The pain and I breathe the same air. And the pain transforms into power.

Compare that to a literal description of what healing feels like: Traumatic experiences taught my brain that other people and my own internal experiences are not safe. But many people and all of my internal experiences *are* safe. I teach my brain this by paying gentle attention to uncomfortable emotions as they happen and noticing that I am not unsafe while those emotions happen.

Such a literal description begs the question: *How* do you "pay gentle attention"? How do you notice you're safe during unsafe-feeling emotions? What does it feel like?

I can't describe it without a metaphor: It feels like I'm on fire, but also I am the ocean, and also I am love. There is no literal description clearer than that. Nothing in our mundane lives can capture the internal experience of healing from trauma, neglect, and abuse.

We need stories of magic to talk about healing from trauma, neglect, and abuse. When you "escape" into a fantasy, maybe you're healing yourself. The importance of processing TNA through fantasy and magical metaphors is why I give whole talks about the parallels between cartoons and the science of emotions and trauma—not just *Moana*, but *Inside Out* (emotion dismissing), *Frozen* (childhood trauma and neglect), *Encanto* (intergenerational trauma), and *Turning Red* (bicultural trauma).

How does trauma heal? Every day, a miracle happens, that's how. We wake up; we carry the Ring. We brush our teeth; we befriend the monster. We live our lives; we talk about Bruno.

Yes, go to therapy and practice self-care and connect with trustworthy people. Practice yoga or tai chi or other body-based experiences of feeling safe inside your skin. Heal in the real world. And self-soothe in a fictional world where your insides can finally match your outsides. There's a reason our stories are full of magic. It's because we survivors are full of magic.

Bodies change with time and experience. Curiosity is often our best, most foolproof tool for approaching these changes. It may not be sufficient, but it's never the wrong place to start.

Chapter 7 tl;dr:

- Curiosity is turning toward what's true, regardless of whether it's what you wish were true or were taught "should" be true, and saying, "I see you. I love you. I want to know you." This, rather than turning toward what's happening with FEAR, RAGE, or PANIC/GRIEF.

- Bodies change and vary over time. Especially with age, illness, or injury, our bodies may have new needs that could alter the ways partners give and receive care in the relationship. As long as you can see your partner as themselves, separate from their needs, you'll maintain a connection that embraces bodies as they are.

- I don't know one person who didn't absorb sexual shame from somewhere, whether it was from their family, their religion, or popular culture. The more we let ourselves notice the shame and shine a light on what it wants to hide, the more of ourselves we make available for connection and pleasure.

- A lot of us carry trauma in our bodies. Beyond therapy and safe connection and practices like yoga, many survivors use stories of magic and fantasy to experience and articulate something that approximates survivorship more accurately than anything in our daily lives.

Some Good Questions:

- In what contexts is it easy to be in a curious space in my mind?

- Where does shame live in my body, emotions, or thoughts? Where does it live in my partner? What would happen if we, as our best selves, spoke to each other of our shame?

- What magic have I developed in response to the trauma, neglect, or abuse I should never have had to endure? What's my superpower? What am I quested to carry? Who is my Samwise? What mythical creatures do my bidding? Am *I* a mythical creature? Can I visit my deceased ancestors to access their wisdom and love? What calls me?

Chapter 8

RELATIONSHIP CHANGE:

Creating It and Coping with It

Two of the most difficult questions I get asked when I teach about the science of sexuality are:

"I like these ideas, but how do I get my partner on board with the changes you're describing?"

"Nothing you're saying will help us until we resolve this old hurt that just will not heal. How do we get past that?"

Both of these questions are, at their core: "How do we change?"

And change is plenty hard when there's just one person involved; but if change requires two people to collaborate? So much more difficult.

Let's notice, before we go any further, that the question is "How do *we* change?" not "How do I change my partner?" or "How do I change for my partner?" Like, "How do I convince my partner to change their mind about planning sex?" or "How do I get my partner to just let go of stuff that happened in the past?"

Unlike relationships we don't expect to last into the distant future, long-term relationships require effective strategies for changing *together*.

I want to show you how partners I know have answered these questions, using the tools we've discussed in the last few chapters. I'll also add some science about how humans create intentional change—specifically: We only change a little at a time, and it's normal for old hurts to keep hurting, even when the hurt has healed.

"How Do I Get My Partner On Board?"

One of the most common questions I get from people who have read *CAYA* or attended a workshop by themselves is "This is great, I can see how it might even be life-changing! But so far my partner has only responded negatively when I've brought it up. How can I get them on board?"

The short answer is: Be curious about where they are right now. You're already normal, and if you turn with calm, warm curiosity toward whatever is happening in your sexual connection, regardless of whether it matches your expectations or not, you're already doing it *perfectly*. There is no urgency; the stakes are low. A long-term relationship is hardly ever at risk because of a sex issue per se; if there's a true threat to a relationship, it's nearly always some other issue that manifests itself in the sexual connection. Save urgency for the problems where you truly have something to lose, like disagreements about money, children, or health issues, which can have immediate and life-altering consequences.

When you want to get your partner on board with a change to your erotic connection, it's often helpful to have a realistic idea of how people change. So let's talk about that.

As neuroendocrinologist Robert Sapolsky puts it, "You can't reason someone out of something they were never reasoned into." Facts might not care about anyone's feelings, but also feelings don't care about anyone's facts. Soliciting your partner's collaboration on some change in your sexual relationship is never a practice in "convincing" them or trying to persuade them. It's never about them being wrong and you being right (or vice versa).

Too often, when we want our partners to change, we have a vision of the change process that goes from A → B, like this: "Today, my partner thinks, feels, or does this old set of reactions; tomorrow, after they listen to me and understand my point of view and agree that I am correct, they will think, feel, or do a new set of actions that align with what I think, feel, or do."

And that is almost never how it works.

Rather than A → B, it's more like A → E, with all the steps in between.[1] In public health jargon, we call it "readiness to change," and "readiness" comes in roughly five "stages": Pre-contemplation, Contemplation, Preparation, Action, and Maintenance.[2]

When you approach a partner to ask for change, to get them on board, rather than trying to get them from A → E all in one step, just aim to get them *one step further* in their readiness. Let's take each stage in turn and consider what helps to move someone one more step.

STAGE 1: PRE-CONTEMPLATION. This person isn't even considering change. You'll hear them use "sustain talk," which is language that indicates that the situation is not worth changing or can't be changed. "Things are fine." "We're too busy to worry about this right now." "We've already tried, let's give it a rest."

Let's normalize pre-contemplation. We spend almost all of our time neither interested in nor ready for change around almost all of our beliefs and behaviors. There is nothing wrong with a person who is not ready for change. Intentional change can be difficult, and our lives are plenty hard without adding more change on top. Indeed, partners who are already on board for change might still not be ready. As the deadline for this book approached, my interest in sex vanished into a black hole of irony. My spouse and I simply accepted that I did not have the wherewithal even to discuss being interested in sex. We looked at the calendar and agreed, "We'll talk about it on this date, after the book is done." Partners who bring a child into their lives can do the same thing. "We will check in again on this topic in X weeks/months."

But if your partner is both uninterested in change and not yet on board, try not to judge their resistance to change. Instead, be curious about it. You might even say things like "I can understand why you wouldn't be interested in even just talking about this," or "If it weren't so impactful on me, I wouldn't want to change either."

When a partner is in pre-contemplation, it's an exercise in trust—being there for your partner, right where they are, without pushing.

You can be there without pushing because, given the luxury of time that comes with a long-term relationship, you can allow change to happen rather than forcing it. Because it's a long-term relationship, by definition you have time to breathe and allow your partner to be where they are.*

If they do not have some basic information that would let them know that their life could be improved if they explored change, you can try offering them that basic information, as in:

"I'm reading this book that says some things I've never considered before about sex in long-term relationships. I don't know how much of it is relevant to us, but can I tell you about an idea that sounds interesting?"

Or "Now might not be the right time for us to try to change anything, but we'd both like things to change someday, so I've been learning a little about the science. If you're interested, I can tell you some of the new things I'm reading."

And in the meantime: admiration. Admiration is often a great place to begin a change conversation—nothing lowers defenses and opens someone's heart to a difficult conversation like authentic praise and gratitude for all the things they do right. In terms of a change conversation, explicit and genuine admiration also enhances your partner's sense of autonomy, reducing any sense of being criticized, which would only increase defensiveness.

STAGE 2: CONTEMPLATION. This person has become interested in change. They're considering what it might be like to change or what steps they might take if they decided to create change. It's

---

* If the relationship is at stake and you can't get your partner on board, the change you're seeking is not really a change in the sex. Time to adapt the question from chapter 1: "What is it that I want when I want this change to our sexual connection?"

often triggered by a specific, major event or by a long accumulation of many minor (to them) events. You'll hear them use "change talk," which is language that shows that change potentially is on the table for them. "That's something we might try in the future." "This is important. I think we could make it happen." "After what happened last week, I feel like we're ready."

To facilitate a partner's transition from pre-contemplation to contemplation, it's helpful to ask questions that amplify the advantages of change and disadvantages of the status quo. We're asking questions rather than explaining, because our goal is to increase our partner's interest in change, not tell them why they *should* be interested.

ADVANTAGES-OF-CHANGE QUESTIONS:

- What would be some good things about . . . ?

- If you could wave a magic wand and make things change immediately, what would change, and how would your life be better?

DISADVANTAGES-OF-THE-STATUS-QUO QUESTIONS:

- What difficulties/hassles/struggles have we had, when it comes to . . . ?

- How has this stopped us from having the life/relationship we want?

- What might happen if we don't change?

STAGE 3: PREPARATION. This person is almost ready for change. They're making plans and taking steps to get ready for change. They may be reading books or articles about the change or initiating conversations with people who've been through similar change. They might perceive themselves as already changing, and to some extent they are! You'll hear planning talk. If you're reading this book, you might be in preparation. If your partner handed you this book, they might want to help you transition from contemplation to preparation. And it's working!

The goal of transitioning from contemplation to preparation is to transform *interest* into *intention*. A conversational approach to helping a partner make the shift is to ask questions that enhance their intention or commitment to change.

INTENTION-TO-CHANGE QUESTIONS:

- How important is this change to you/us?

- What might you/we be willing to try?

- If you/we were going to make a plan for change, what would it be? (The "if" here respects the other person's autonomy; you are not forcing them to plan, you're simply contemplating a hypothetical plan together.)

STAGE 4: ACTION. This person is actively creating change, altering behavior patterns, adjusting and adapting to a new reality. You're not just reading about responsive desire, you're adjusting your bedroom (like the way my partner and I made a sex towel drawer). You're not just talking about the emotional floorplan, you're actually mapping yours and helping each other transition into spaces closer to the LUST space.

To facilitate a partner's transition from preparation to action, it's helpful to ask questions that amplify your shared confidence in the change.

OPTIMISM-ABOUT-CHANGE QUESTIONS:

- How confident are we that we could create change, if we chose to?

- What personal strengths do we have that will help us succeed?

- Who can offer us support? What steps do we take, if we feel stuck?

At this stage in the change process: admiration, admiration, admiration! Look at you go! Even when you try things that don't work out, *you're doing it*! You're exploring new things, experimenting, playing together! Say your admiration for your partner and your relationship out loud. Heck, *I* admire you for getting this far!

STAGE 5: MAINTENANCE. This person has changed and is actively using their new skills and awareness to sustain that change across new and varied situations. To help a partner transition from action to maintenance, keep communication open with consistent, mutual feedback about the change.

FEEDBACK-ABOUT-CHANGE QUESTIONS:

- What's working?

- What's your favorite thing about the change?

- Is anything not working? What could be better?

Apply the sex-positive definition of "perfect" here. This new pattern you've established may not be everything you had in mind when you began, but you're still within the cycle of woundedness to healing, and wherever you are in the cycle is perfect.[3]

Intentional change happens when (and only when) people are ready, willing, and able to change. Sometimes, though, the energy people bring to the "How do I get my partner on board?" question is "My needs are not being met and I urgently require my partner to change so that my needs will be met." Since your urgency doesn't change the reality that your partner will need time and help to transition into the change, you can manage your feelings by being curious about them. Return to that scenic viewpoint on your emotional floorplan and observe your urgent need for change, without judgment and without buying into it.

The great thing about long-term relationships, in which you've decided to stay together till death do you part and stuff, is that you have time for the situation to change gradually. The situation was probably created gradually, settling into its current state after months or years. Changing the situation may also take months or years. When the change feels too urgent for patience, be curious about the urgency. What's really at stake if things don't change more quickly?

Mike and Kendra

Kendra and Mike were trying to move away from a focus on desire and instead focus on co-creating a context that emphasized pleasure. They went to a sex coach who used an approach called "Motivational Interviewing," which leverages the stages of change, accepting where people are and fully supporting their autonomy. It promotes thinking about change without creating pressure or expectation to change. After establishing some simple ground rules, here's what that conversation sounded like (with the bickering edited out for simplicity):

COACH: *Let's start by making sure coaching is a good fit for you, rather than therapy. Is your relationship at stake here? Would either of you end the relationship if your sexual connection doesn't change?*

M & K: *Oh, no. Definitely not. We love each other, we want to be together, we value each other as people, as co-parents, as friends. We've lived with this for so long, a few more years won't change that.*

COACH: *Okay. So you're here because you're interested in exploring change, but no matter what happens, at least for the middle-term future, neither of you is in so much distress that you'd be motivated to end the relationship. Is that right?*

M & K: *Yes, and actually it's nice to remember that and to be assured of it by each other.*

COACH: *Fantastic. So let's start by making a list. What are some of the good things about where you are right now, in terms of your sexual connection?*

M & K: *Uh . . .*

COACH: *Would it be easier to start with some not-so-good things about where you are right now?*

M & K: *Yes. We're not having sex very often and we've been fighting about how often we have sex since our preschooler was a fetus. That frustration leaks out into other parts of our lives, like a kind of generalized resentment and frustration and dissatisfaction. It's harder to appreciate each other when it feels like everything is somehow tied to whether or not we're having sex. And it's so easy to resent each other over small things, when what we're actually resenting is this permanent—not permanent, just long-standing—battle. It's like it's transformed from being about sex to being about power and who's right and who's being listened to and taken seriously. Also, Mike feels really lonely without the sex and Kendra feels really guilty about it, but also we both feel resentful. Very, very resentful.*

COACH: *Okay. Good list! If you think of other things we can always add to it. How about some good things, though? Some good things about where you are now?*

M & K: *We do actually have sex sometimes, and we both enjoy it. Sometimes it's amazing! We also like how we feel after we have sex that we had because we both were into it, compared to the sex we have when Kendra is just doing it out of obligation or guilt. It actually does nice things for us as a couple when we're connecting sexually, we feel closer.*

COACH: *Okay. Another great list! When you look at these*

two lists side by side like this, what do you notice? What do you see?

M & K: *Well, there's more stuff on the not-so-good side. It looks like the problem really is the lack of feeling nurtured and supported, the guilt, and maybe above all the resentment. There's so many hurt feelings for both of us.*

COACH: *And when you think about all of this, what are some strategies you might use—and maybe there are strategies you're already using—to get the good stuff and maybe minimize some of this not-so-good stuff?*

M & K: *We really need to address the mutual resentment, which has grown so far beyond just sex. And we have to keep trying to focus on how much pleasure we experience when we do—that's something we're doing right.*

COACH: *It's pretty hard to create a context that facilitates pleasure while you're still carrying all that resentment around in your bodies. And Mike, you might have to heal your resentment without first getting the sex you've been longing for.*

M & K: *Oof, this is . . . a project.*

COACH: *Yes, okay, good work so far. So if you were going to create change, to get all this good stuff and minimize some of the not-so-good stuff, it sounds like you might try addressing each person's resentment outside of a sexual context, and, in parallel, try increasing pleasure, also outside of a sexual context. Does that sound right?*

M & K: *[nod in agreement]*

With the help of the coach, Mike and Kendra developed a hypothetical plan, including the number of times per week that they would have tough conversations to seriously address the resentment, and the number of times per week they would create time and space to share nonsexual pleasure. They established some potential ground rules for how those times would go.

COACH: *Okay! Now you have these lists and you have some hypothetical plans. The goal at this point in the process is to choose a simple, really doable plan over which you both feel equal ownership and responsibility. Aim for small changes right now that will give you a lot of success. Can we agree on one more thing?*

M & K: *Sure.*

COACH: *Kendra is not the diagnosed patient in this situation. Both of you are equally right and healthy and neither is wrong or broken. What's broken is the connection between you. And repairing the connection will require both of you to invest equally in breaking down this wall of difficult feelings you've built up between you.*

M & K: *. . . Oof.*

This is one example of how couples can think pragmatically about difficult situations like this by talking about the feelings and problems, without being in *the feelings and problems. You take them all out and dump them on the table like puzzle pieces, and you begin sorting. In real life a conversation like this takes a few hours, often spread out over multiple sessions. What matters most is that each person's autonomy is respected, so that no one feels railroaded into anything and no one feels their needs are being neglected. With kindness, patience, and, when necessary, professional support, you can make plans together to get the good stuff and minimize the not-so-good stuff. That's how couples collaborate to co-create a context that makes pleasure easier to access.*

Healing Old Hurts

A special characteristic of a long-term relationship is that both partners will inflict wounds on each other over the years and decades, usually accidentally, occasionally deliberately. Therapists know that this is a normal, all-but-inevitable experience in a long-term relationship. A sex therapist friend of mine described the situation this way:

> *When people are so intimately intwined for such a long period of time, they have access to their partner's most vulnerable points. Maybe they were cheated on, maybe their partner said something cruel in a bad moment, maybe they said something that was meant to be helpful but instead cut deep into an old wound. Both parties want to stay together, they do love each other, they want to have a good sexual connection again, but in those intimate moments the old pain rears up and shuts down the ability to open up sexually. Even if the hurt is not caused intentionally or maliciously, and even after genuine, heartfelt apologies are made and accepted, once that vulnerable spot has been hit, how does the wounded partner let go of that hurt?*

Let me be honest: Healing old hurts is not easy for most couples. It's a collaborative process you cultivate over time, as you accumulate old hurts and you mutually acknowledge that they have to be dealt with or else your relationship will begin to erode. If you can't deal with old hurts around nonsexual issues in your relationship, you'll probably really struggle when it comes to old sexual hurts. Still experiencing flare-ups about that time your partner spent the money you were supposed to be saving, and they didn't tell you? Work on that first, then deal with the time one of you went further than you mutually agreed was acceptable with another partner, or the time someone said something hurtful about the other person's body, sexual history, or ability to give and receive pleasure.

You can use the skills I describe here to work on those other is-sues, then approach a sex-related hurt. Talking about sex can be more difficult than talking about other topics, because we were raised to feel both inherently flawed when it comes to sex and, at the same time, existentially mandated to be excellent at sex.

Let's use two examples, one with a completely non-sex-related old hurt—a physical injury—and one with a sex-related old hurt—an emotional injury. The two are exact parallels, and the more we treat emotional wounds the way we treat physical wounds, the easier it is to avoid blame, shame, resentment, and a sense of helplessness.

First example: When we were kids, maybe eight years old, I hit my sister in the face with a baseball bat. She was standing behind me, playing catcher, as I prepared for our brother's pitch by enthu-siastically swinging the bat over my shoulder.

Wham.

I split her lip and knocked out both of her front teeth.[4]

It was an accident.* I felt remorseful. I apologized. None of that changed the fact of her injury. My apology could not stop her lip from bleeding and her face from bruising; my remorse could not end the pain; the fact that it was an accident could not make her teeth grow in. Only time and wound care could do that. In the meantime—over a year, as it happened—she had to live without her front teeth.

Amelia will never again stand behind me while I'm holding a baseball bat, not because she hasn't forgiven me or because she thinks I did it on purpose, but because her brain very reasonably sends a red alert signal if it notices me with a bat in my hands. And in fact, I haven't voluntarily held a baseball bat in the vicinity of my sister since that day. This is the crucial parallel with emotional wounds: Though the injury itself has healed, it leaves traces in our brains' alert systems—in both the person who was hurt and the person who regrets causing the harm.

It's pretty easy to view a physical injury with OBSERVATIONAL DISTANCE, with nonjudgment. No one judges Amelia's lip for not

---

* All the examples I'll use are of *accidental* harm. If the old, lingering hurt you're dealing with was intentional, that brings up additional trust issues, so therapy may be worth considering.

healing because I apologized, and no one judges Amelia's brain for hesitating to stand near me if I'm holding a bat.

Similarly, if I see Amelia avoid me when I'm holding a bat, no judgment on me for feeling remorse all over again, or shame at having hurt my sister, or defensiveness or an amorphous frustration that the old harm still resonates into the present . . . though my friends would tell me there's no need for that ongoing remorse.

Second example: My friends Jamie and Rowan (not their real names) had been married over ten years, together for nearly twenty, when Jamie accidentally criticized Rowan's body. Rowan was sitting on the bed as they got up in the morning, and Jamie, with loving, affectionate intentions, leaned over, grabbed the sides of Rowan's belly, and said, "Beamy!"

"Beamy," like the width of a ship, a broad-beamed ship. Jamie grew up with "the family yacht" money and competed on his college's sailing team, so for him, nautical terms are a love language. He truly meant it lovingly; he told me later he meant to communicate his pride in his partner's body peace. Rowan's "beam" was hard-won, after all. A nonbinary person assigned the "It's a girl!" handbook at birth (more on that in chapter 10), Rowan had a painful history with body dysmorphia and disordered eating, which is even more common among trans and nonbinary people than cisgender people,[5] and Rowan is of a generation when gender divergence was virtually unaddressed in eating disorder treatment, so their struggle was long and isolating. They had lived a lot of their life with intense depression. It had taken years of emotional work and immersion in a queer community to allow them to have a healthy relationship with food. From that healthy, even joyful relationship with food was born . . . their belly. Rowan had, on one occasion, described that belly as a trophy for practicing self-compassion.

But.

It did not matter that Jamie meant it lovingly. Confronted with the word, along with Jamie's hands right on that long-contested part of their body, all the body issues Rowan had ever had in their life rushed to the surface.

It was entirely unintentional, just as me clocking my sister in the face was unintentional. Like me, Jamie saw the pain he caused, and he felt remorse. He apologized, sincerely; that's important, but his remorse and his apology couldn't heal Rowan's hurt, just as mine couldn't heal my sister's lip. What healed Rowan's hurt was the same as what healed my sister's hurt: time and emotional wound care. And in the meantime, Rowan had to live with the wound.

But even with great care, even when the wound has healed, Rowan's brain retains traces of red alert, so that when the couple approaches a sexual context, Rowan's brain tells them to brace for impact. If they're in a particularly vulnerable place emotionally, a mere gesture in the direction of the old injury can fully activate the pain, fresh as if it were the day of the original incident.

And when Jamie notices Rowan withdrawing, or if Rowan says, "I'm having a boat moment," Jamie's brain activates a similar red alert, the shame or defensiveness or amorphous frustration that the harm continues to resonate into the present. The red alerts hit the brakes.

No judgment on Jamie for feeling remorse when he sees Rowan's hesitation, though friends would tell him there's no need for ongoing remorse.

Got it? Pain resonates into the present not necessarily because a wound is unhealed but because our brains learn to fear situations that were harmful in the past.

The first step to unlearning those fears is *nonjudgment*, both for the time it takes to heal and for the residual red alerts that remain in the wake of harm.

From there, you begin the first skill I want to teach here: the Third Thing Conversation.

The old hurt is a third thing—it's not a problem that exists inside one partner, it's a shared project, external to each individual and the relationship.

Let's take the baseball bat example. Suppose some Labor Day weekend, I visit Amelia and a bunch of us decide to play softball in the backyard. Suppose I pick up a bat when it's my turn.

Amelia's body flares with recognition and her brain responds with a small red alert of FEAR.

"Y'all keep your distance from Emily, she's got a bat!" Amelia calls to the family. It's a joke, she's joking, obviously.

And I laugh, because what happened was in the past, it was an accident, her adult teeth grew in, it's fine. But my body flares with recognition of the old hurt and my brain responds with a small red alert of PANIC/GRIEF.

This is all normal; old emotional junk often arises among family members, decades after the original incident. Often, family members can shake it off, let it go, or, if they're old-school, pick themselves up, dust themselves off, and start all over again. Family, yay!

But sometimes we can't. Suppose the red alerts in our brains interfered with our ability to enjoy the holiday. Because Amelia and I have worked hard on our sisterhood and friendship, we might sit down together at the end of the day and talk about the third thing that is our mutual red alerts, to liberate ourselves from them.

Here's my master's degree in counseling, interpreting the conversation we would have:

> EMILY: (Names her feeling) When you joked about the bat, I was reminded of the time I caused you harm, and it felt uncomfortable to remember that I have harmed you in the past.
>
> AMELIA: (Names her feeling) I made the joke because seeing the bat reminded me of the harm you caused. I felt uncomfortable and tried to displace the discomfort. We are both doing our best with the resources available to each of us.
>
> Calm, warm curiosity
>
> EMILY: (Separates the feeling from the past) The event is resolved, yet the emotion lingers, decades later. Still, the fact that I can share that with you is, in itself, healing.

> AMELIA: *(Soothes the feeling) I agree, and it helps that we both know how to move all the way through the tunnel of a difficult feeling to get to the light at the end. We can do that together.*
> EMILY: *(Closes with a tool) I'm grateful we can stay connected, even when it's uncomfortable.*

Nobody talks like that, right? But this is actually how we, as identical twins on the spectrum, talk to each other:

> EMILY: *(Names her feeling) I had a feeling when you joked about the bat.*
> AMELIA: *(Names her feeling) Yeah. I made the joke because I had a feeling.*

> *Calm, warm curiosity*

> EMILY: *(Separates the feeling from the past) Feelings are boring.*
> AMELIA: *(Soothes the feeling) And exhausting.*
> EMILY: *(Closes with a tool—I choose emotional engagement) Boring and exhausting.*

Most people's real conversations will be somewhere between the two extremes of therapy-speak, where everything is explicit, and twin-speak, where everything is spoken in shorthand incomprehensible to others. But there's a basic structure with important elements that make a Third Thing Conversation effective:

> PERSON 1: *Names the difficult feeling they're experiencing, puts it on the table*
> PERSON 2: *Names their difficult feeling (maybe about Person 1's difficult feeling?), puts it on the table.*

> *Both turn toward these difficult feelings with calm, warm curiosity.*

PERSON 1: *Notices that these feelings exist despite the original situation being fully resolved.*

PERSON 2: *Offers a way out of the difficult feelings, unrelated to the original situation, which has already been resolved. (You can return to your answers to the questions about your adverse spaces, to recall the strategies you already know help you move out of them.)*

PERSON 1: *Expresses a blend of admiration, trust, confidence, and joy, and the cycle of woundedness to healing—in short, uses a relationship tool or sex-positive mindset to close the conversation on an unambiguously positive note.*

Here's a similar kind of conversation between me and my spouse, about the reemergence of my low sexual interest. In this instance, I'd been feeling highly self-critical for a number of days, and I finally shared it, knowing that I needed his help to get through this tunnel and find my way to the light:

ME: *(Names her feeling) Is this an okay time to complain a little bit about how rarely we're having sex? I mean, I realize I'm the problem and I'm complaining about how my own stress is getting in the way of sex, but it really does frustrate me that I can't get out of it.*

HIM: *(Names his feeling) You're not a problem and yeah, I don't like your stress either, and not just because of the sex. I hate seeing you unhappy.*

Calm, warm curiosity

ME: *(Separates the feeling from the past) You know it's not about you. I love you and I'm attracted to you and I want to be interested, I'm just . . . my brain just can't.*

> HIM: *(Soothes the feeling) You wanna order takeout and watch* A Mighty Wind?
>
> ME: *(Closes with a tool—I choose admiration)* HOW DID YOU KNOW???

Our conversation didn't sound this straightforward. I've mentioned before that my spouse's attention moves fast, so there were a lot of tangents and some "What ifs?" about other situations. It's my role in these serious conversations to return us to our task. Early in our relationship, I was frustrated by this, but I learned quickly that I can have any conversation, discuss any difficult topic, go to the deepest, darkest, scariest emotional places, if I just accept that I'm walking through the tunnel with a very excited puppy. He bounces all over, while I keep us moving forward . . . and he's the one who finds the light first and guides me to it. Your conversations may be similarly messy and tangential. All that matters is that you keep the problem as a third thing, not something innate to one or the other of you.

My friends Jamie and Rowan are also really great at communicating, but they had a pattern to overcome. They had taken some great advice from a therapist: Don't bring it up in the moment. If the old hurt arises, wait until you're calm to discuss it, so that you don't argue while you're already activated with stress. That's generally a great approach. However, as a consequence of it, if the old pain arose when they started to have sex, they either didn't have sex or else—oof—Rowan went ahead and had the sex while also feeling the bad feelings.

But after years of talking about it outside the feeling, the old hurt was still popping up and hitting the brakes, especially when Jamie tried to initiate sex, and both of them were frustrated that all their careful processing hadn't gotten rid of it.

So I said, "Talk about it in the moment. When you start feeling it, pause the sex and process the feeling—not to stop the sex, but so that you can eliminate the ambivalence and have sex worth having." I told them my Coen story, the time I paused things to inquire about potential unwanted consequences, and how, yes, talking about it shifted the experience of desire, but then we could have playful, pleasurable sex without the ambivalence.

It did not work the first time they tried, or even the first few times. It was too difficult to move through the feelings, and they ended up cuddling instead of having the sex they planned.

FORGIVENESS: HOW TO

According to scientists, forgiveness means something like the absence of negative thoughts, feelings, and behaviors toward the transgressor, and perhaps the presence of positive thoughts, feelings, and behaviors toward them.[6]

In real life, people mean lots of different things when they use the word "forgiveness." Is forgiveness the mere statement of: "I forgive you"? Is it getting to a place where you no longer invest your energy in negative thoughts and emotions about the person who caused you harm? Is it the re-acceptance of the forgiven person into your life? Do you necessarily trust a person you forgive?

In my opinion, forgiveness is whatever forgiveness is for you. Forgiveness doesn't even have to be a choice you make or an action you take. As I always say, difficult feelings are tunnels. You go all the way through the darkness to get to the light at the end; forgiveness can simply be the place you find yourself when you get to the end of the tunnel.

Be sure to notice if someone asks for forgiveness and you say, "I forgive you," but they're not satisfied. They want more than the forgiveness they got. Maybe they want to restore your relationship to what it was before. Maybe they want to hear you say they didn't do anything wrong in the first place. Maybe they want to know that you love them just the same. None of these things has to be included with your forgiveness, though any of them may be.

"I forgive you and I never want to see you again" can be forgiveness.

"I forgive you for the wrong you did and the harm you caused" can be forgiveness, too.

"I forgive you and I don't think our love will ever be the same" can be forgiveness.

And "I forgive you, and our relationship is better because we went through this struggle together" can be forgiveness.

Forgiveness doesn't mean the old hurt never comes up again—and the worst thing to do when someone who has forgiven you is once again experiencing the hurt, is to say, "But you forgave me!"

Forgiveness is like love. When you love someone, it simply means you love them. When you forgive someone, it simply means you forgive them for harm they caused. Whether your relationship is still intact is a separate question.

Something to notice about the third thing, curiosity-based approach to dealing with old hurts: No one says, "But I already apologized, what else do you want?" You have successfully decoupled the hurt from the resolved incident. Today's discomfort is not about the past incident, and therefore it's not about who apologized or how. The Third Thing Conversation is about being there for the uncomfortable feelings happening right now.

My favorite thing about Rowan and Jamie's story is that the moment they made major progress broke the "rules" I've been describing. It happened when they turned *against* the third thing. It went something like this:

ROWAN: *(Names their feeling)* [*inarticulate groan into Jamie's chest*]
JAMIE: *(Names his feeling) Not again.*

Calm, warm curiosity

ROWAN: *(Separates the feeling from the past) I'm not even . . . I'm literally just bored at this point. I'm fucking bored of having to deal with this shit. I'm bored trying to be compassionate toward the feeling. Fuck that, I don't love the feeling, I hate the feeling, I'm done with it. Fuck off, feeling!*
JAMIE: *(Soothes the feeling) Fuck off, feeling! We're done with you!*
ROWAN: *(Closes with a tool) I'm gonna fucking show this feeling. You think you can ruin sex? Not today, Satan. I'm gonna lie spread eagle on this bed with the lights on and love the shit out of my body until I come so hard I can't walk. Get on it, babe.*

The second skill for healing old hurts is something I call the "What If?" Daydream.

The tragedy of old hurts is that you can never go back and undo them, however much you might wish you could . . . or can you?

Allow me to introduce you to the "What If?" Daydream.

With a "What If?" Daydream, you reimagine the hurt, imagine it vividly and viscerally, and you imagine for yourself exactly what you needed in that moment of distress. Don't imagine that the hurt never happened, just imagine that someone had been there for you in an ideal way, fully present, utterly safe and loving, holding you until the pain got a little easier. What if you had been safe in that moment? In the language of the floorplan, the question is: What if, the instant the harm happened, all the adverse spaces in your floorplans disappeared and all you could access were the favorable spaces of SEEKING, PLAY, LUST, and above all CARE?

Can imagining a different past create real emotional healing in the present? Sure it can! It's our imaginations that activate the red alert signal, in anticipation of a potential risk. If our imagination can activate a physiological stress response, that means it can activate a physiological healing response. If you were dealing with physical pain, we might call this kind of fantasy a "corrective experience," training your brain to feel safe in the presence of pain. But it works for emotional pain, too.

As an example, let's start with my sister's front teeth and her avoidance of me with a bat. She and I would sit together, and she could daydream aloud:

AMELIA: *What if, when you hit me in the face, we already had a perfect caregiver with us? What if our grandmother, as her ideal self, had been there with hugs and a first aid kit and all the compassion in the world? (This would be especially powerful because our grandmother died twenty years ago, so we're invoking an ancestor who brings the power of infinite wisdom and kindness.)*

EMILY: *What if she had been there and used the opportunity to teach me to tend to wounds, so that I could be a part of the caregiving? She'd tell me to run and get ice, and she'd show me how to put it in a washcloth and press it to the wound to stop the bleeding.*

AMELIA: *And we would both be allowed to cry as much as we needed to, and once my mouth stopped hurting she would feed us her breaded chicken with cheese sauce, which is the most perfect food anyone ever tasted.*

EMILY: *Then we would make dessert with the Snoopy Sno-cone Machine she got for us even though we didn't keep our room clean for a whole month. It would feel good on your gums.*

Even a decades-old harm can benefit from a reimagined, ideal "What If?" Daydream.

Let's apply the daydream to our couple with the hurtful body image comment. They sat on the couch together and tried it:

> ROWAN: *What if, in the moment after you said those words, you were gifted with psychic abilities, and you could instantly and fully understand all the ways I was impacted? Imagine if I didn't have to do all that explaining, you just knew, in an instant, about the hurts and insecurity that already lived inside me and the ways your words just echoed down across all of that pain.*
>
> JAMIE: *And what if, because I understood right then all the ways you were suffering, I was suddenly a perfect caregiver, fully trustworthy and knowing exactly what to say and do? Imagine that I had no defensiveness and no guilt, just unlimited love for you. What if I knew exactly the words that would heal those wounds—not just the one from my words, but all those old wounds from your childhood and especially the ones from high school. Imagine I could hold you and say exactly the right words.*

Now, it might have been the case that Rowan suddenly knew exactly the right words, like maybe "I love your body because it's part of you, and that has nothing to do with how it looks." And Jamie could have said that and meant it. But Rowan didn't know the words, so they let the details be vague, even when the emotional experience was specific and intense:

> ROWAN: *You say exactly the right words, and my body hears them and believes them.*

Imagining a past that could never have happened, they actually created the experience right there on the sofa. They held each other and cried.

The "What If?" Daydream is for people who are ready to imagine a reality that could never have existed in the moment but is, nevertheless, a reality that we can co-create in our shared memory. My sister and I imagined a "what if" that could have actually happened, but Rowan and Jamie imagined magic for themselves. "What if we had magic?" is a gorgeous use of the "What If?" Daydream, because our imaginations aren't limited to the real world. Just as magical metaphors can help trauma survivors to understand their survivorship, "What If?" Daydreams can resolve unfinished emotional business with resources that don't exist in real life. It's a shared *daydream,* not a wish for the past to be different.

When I used this practice with my spouse, we imagined that our present-day selves could go back and tell our eight-years-ago selves what we know now. We didn't say, "If only I had known then what I know now," we said, "What if I could go back and tell myself everything I've learned since then?" We told each other what we would tell our past selves, and just like that, we felt as if our past selves knew what we had learned and could be at peace.

In her book *I Hope We Choose Love: A Trans Girl's Notes from the End of the World,* writer and healer Kai Cheng Thom acknowledges the deep bullshit in which our lives are mired, and offers a soul-warming, optimistic, and utterly practical solution: Choose love. If you're angry, you have every right to be. Hold your anger with love. If you're despairing, you have every right to be. Hold your despair with love.

The "hold" of love is not a tight fist but an open palm. Hold your anger, your despair, your loneliness, your fear, in the palms of your hands, like a bird or a palmful of water from a stream or an offering of rose petals. Observe them with calm, warm curiosity. Show them to your partner so they, too, can witness your pain with calm, warm curiosity. Witness the difficult feelings from your internal space of OBSERVATIONAL DISTANCE.

Sometimes your partner comes to you with their anger, despair, loneliness, or fear held tenderly in the palms of their hands.

If your partner is angry, they have every right to be. Hold their anger with love. If your partner is despairing, they have every right to be. Hold their despair with love. Hello, anger. Hello, despair. I see you. I love you. I want to know you.

The tools discussed in this chapter can help you and a partner collaborate on your shared garden. But maybe they feel too complicated, difficult, or out of reach. If that's you, I want to talk to you about the biggest, meanest barriers between you and the long-term sexual connection you're longing for. Regardless of your relationship structure or the genders of the people involved or your ages or anything else, you were raised in a culture full of people who had *opinions,* and they very much expect you to agree with those opinions and organize your life around them. We'll use all the tools and science we've described so far to overcome this barrier made of other people's opinions. I think of it as two parts: the sex imperatives and the gender mirage. They're the topics of the next two chapters.

Chapter 8 tl;dr:

- Intentional change happens gradually. It can be cultivated, but never forced. People don't change faster because we get more impatient with them.

- How you approach a partner with a change should be shaped by where they are in their readiness to change: pre-contemplation, contemplation, preparation, action, or maintenance. You can facilitate change *one step at a time.*

- In any relationship that lasts long enough, partners will experience emotional wounds that persist long after the incidents that caused them are over. They heal the way physical injuries heal: with time and care. Apologies and remorse are important, but they can't knit a person back together. Instead, what works is turning toward the old wound as a third thing, a shared project that partners want to heal together.

- These old injuries last because of the fear we associate with the original injury, rather than because of ongoing harm. Our well-intentioned imagination makes the pain linger; that means we can use our imaginations to free ourselves from the fear, through a "What If?" Daydream.

Some Good Questions:

- If my partner wanted me to make a change, how would I want them to approach me?

- What is it that each of us wants from change? How will we know when enough change has happened?

- What genuinely is at stake when it comes to creating change? Would a partner leave the relationship if the situation isn't resolved to their satisfaction?

- Can we separate solving the problem itself from the process of dealing with all the feelings each person has about the problem? Might we even start feeling better about each other before we've finished creating the change we want? What do our floorplans tell us works to help each person move through the adverse spaces into positive spaces?

Chapter 9

THE SEX IMPERATIVES

In their book, *Magnificent Sex,* Peggy Kleinplatz and A. Dana Ménard describe their interviews with people of many sexual orientations, gender identities, and ages, kinky and vanilla, and monogamous or in open relationships, who had one thing in common: They self-identified as having *extraordinary* sex lives. In the interviews, researchers inquired not just about what extraordinary sex was like, but also how each person had found their way to the experience.

Answer? First "Unlearning," meaning "unlearning much of what they previously thought they knew about sex and sexuality," including "negative, destructive or simply constricting messages." The second answer was "Letting Go and Overcoming," meaning they had to "deconstruct and overcome the restrictive ideas about sex and themselves that had become embedded in their minds."

These negative messages and restrictive ideas are the lies I talked about in chapter 5. They're false beliefs that might make sexual difficulties feel urgent and high-stakes, as if you have so much to lose if you don't "fix" your sex life. These messages can also make the tools and mindsets I've described so far feel out of reach or impossible to apply.

Crucially, every participant who had experienced these negative influences (and nearly all participants had) overcame them and went on to become a person who had magnificent sex.

You can, too.

In this chapter I want to discuss what some of those negative or limiting ideas might be, along with two important strategies for unearthing these weeds, to get them out of your erotic gardens for good.

The Sex Imperatives

In chapter 1, I mentioned a queer Gen X woman who felt that her need to be desired stemmed from a part of her that was convinced she was unfuckable—this, despite the fact that she was actually doing a lot of fucking at the time.

Why couldn't all that fucking convince this part of her that she was fuckable?

She said, "The feeling of unfuckability is not about fucking at all. It's actually about cultural validation. It's about feeling seen and valued as a sex object, seeing yourself reflected in the culture as a sex object. There was nobody that looked like me in movies or TV being portrayed as fuckable. So it didn't matter who I fucked because I was confusing actual fucking for cultural validation."

"When I talk to other people," I replied, "sometimes they connect fuckability to lovability, a feeling of belonging. Like, to feel unfuckable is to feel that you're out in the cold and will never be allowed inside."

"Yes!" she said.

"So . . . that's an attachment wound," I said, referring to the PANIC/GRIEF space.

"My dad left when I was little!" she affirmed.

"So this wound when you were little met a culture that said the way to be safe from abandonment was to be sexually desirable, and that culture was also saying—"

"That I wasn't that," she finished. "Yes."

This is just one example of the ways our imperfect childhoods become toxic when, at adolescence (or sooner), they meet a culture of sexual "imperatives." These imperatives define not just who gets to be sexual, but how sex should happen. In *Mediated Intimacy: Sex Advice in Media Culture*, Meg-John Barker, Rosalind Gill, and Laura Harvey document the ubiquitous imperatives in sex advice in mainstream media like women's magazines and TV shows. Do any of these sound familiar?

- The "coital imperative" to have penis-in-vagina sex (since heterosexuality is just assumed)

- The "variety imperative" to have manual, oral, and anal play, in addition to penis-in-vagina sex

- The "performance imperative," to enhance your sexual skill set like an ambitious employee pursuing a promotion, "to work on and discipline the body" and "make time to work at sex"

And more: the "confidence imperative," the "pleasure imperative," the imperative to have a relationship "because sex is better within an intimate relationship," and the "sex imperative" itself, to be a sexual person who wants and has and even likes sex.

To this list, I add the "monogamy imperative," because you should have only one sexual relationship (at a time), and the "desire imperative," which I described in chapter 2—the imperative to experience spontaneous desire on a regular basis, regardless of the context.

We can also list any number of body imperatives, what my friend would describe as the "fuckabilty imperative," to conform as closely as you can to a culturally constructed (and highly gendered) aesthetic ideal, and to work relentlessly to discipline your body, never to accept your body as it is.

Where do we get these ideas about the sex imperatives? From *everywhere*. They're in explicit sex advice, sure, but also in movies and TV, in porn, and even in what our friends are willing to talk about. People read romance novels and erotica as "scripts" or even self-help for improving their sex lives. Could the wild popularity of the *Fifty Shades* phenomenon be partly explained because women read it as a potential script to access the sexual satisfaction they'd been missing? Some people certainly did.[1] A therapist at a workshop I led said she was working with a couple who treated *Fifty Shades* as a textbook and she was conflicted because it seemed to her that "BDSM seems inherently abusive." Particularly worrying to me was that even the therapist thought *Fifty Shades* was an accurate representation of BDSM and therefore she thought BDSM was inevitably coercive.

Readers in the BDSM community will be relieved to know that my answer was "Oh golly no! No! *Fifty Shades* is not BDSM! There are so many other, better books they could be reading!"[2]

The imperatives are sometimes incredibly specific in their ideas about what happens during sex. For example, a straight couple were engaged but wanted to solve a sexual difficulty before they fully committed to marriage, so they went to therapy. The problem was he wanted her to swallow his ejaculate when she went down on him, and she did not want to swallow.

They used an approach like the approach in chapter 1: What did he want when he wanted her to swallow? What did she not want when she didn't want to swallow?

He wanted to feel fully accepted, he said. To have the experience of a blow job that didn't end with her mouth leaving his penis, but staying through the entire process.

And she didn't like how her digestion felt afterward, for one thing. Also, she did not want to feel pressured to do something she didn't like.

Solution: How might they feel about him ejaculating in her mouth but her not swallowing? Just leave it there on his genitals afterward, or maybe even kiss him and transfer the ejaculate to his mouth to swallow (sometimes called "snowballing")?

Yep. That got them both what they wanted and avoided the things they didn't want. He was not interested in having his own ejaculate in his mouth, but he was on board with ejaculating in her mouth and her not swallowing.

I learned of this couple through their therapist—a marriage and family therapist, not a sex therapist. When I suggested to her that the couple talk through pros and cons and maybe find a compromise like this one, the therapist told me it had never occurred to either client or even to her that someone could allow a partner to ejaculate into their mouth and then *not* swallow. Sometimes when I tell this story, people can't understand how neither the therapist nor either partner had ever heard of "spit or swallow." This shows how much people can vary in the sexual imperatives they've absorbed from the culture.

Sometimes people's unspoken, subconscious sex imperatives make it difficult for me even to understand their questions. At a workshop in a sex toy store, an attendee had to rephrase their question three times before I realized they were assuming that "anal play" always meant penetration.

When I finally caught on, I said, "Oh, I see! Yeah, no, when I say 'anal play,' I'm talking about any and all anal play, and most of that is external. You don't have to push your tongue into your partner's anus in order to do anilingus, you can just kiss or lick around the external part of the sphincter and perineum, and when you touch with your fingers, again, no penetration needs to be involved . . . though, still definitely try adding lube to your fingers, even for external touch."

"Ohhhhh," said the workshop attendee.

And then we talked about managing involuntary tension of the anal sphincter.

The tools from part 1—especially calm, warm curiosity and the adjusted definitions of "normal" and "perfect"—are intended to help you address situations when a sex imperative shows up in your sex life and you decide to address it directly.

But the challenge with unspoken assumptions is that they're unspoken. You may not even realize they're there, the way the couple in therapy didn't realize they were assuming that if someone ejaculates in your mouth, your only option is to swallow it. The workshop attendee didn't notice that they were assuming if they agreed to anal play they were agreeing to anal penetration.

You always have another option. To swallow or not. To kiss or not. To orgasm or not. To keep going or to stop. To ask your partner to change something or to let them keep doing what they're doing. You can use words to express what you want and like; you can use nonverbal vocalization; you can use body language. *You get to choose.*

Ama and Di

My friends do not always take my advice. No matter how often I said, "Other people's sex lives have nothing to do with yours," Di wanted to know how often a typical couple has sex, according to the research.

Her reason? Di was haunted by the idea of "lesbian bed death."

"Lesbian bed death" is the idea that sex eventually evaporates in long-term sexual relationships between women.

And look, it just doesn't.[3] I mean, it may have in your personal experience, just as it may in any relationship. But lesbians are not more likely to experience "bed death" than anyone else.

But Di looked up the average frequency of sex, the measure of central tendency that doesn't mean anything useful, and, inevitably, reflexively, compared their sex life to that completely irrelevant number . . . and she was suddenly really worried that they were "doing it wrong."

What I love about this story is that simple facts went a long way in solving the problem. This is a rare circumstance that I cherish in my nerdy heart.

I didn't quite assemble a PowerPoint presentation about the research, but I did announce to them that I would like, in the words of lesbian sex therapist Suzanne Iasenza, to put this myth "to bed." I gave them this summary of what's actually true about sex in long-term lesbian relationships: Lesbian partners are more likely to report having sex less frequently as the relationship goes on, or possibly at every stage of the relationship. But they also report:

- *Having very similar levels of sexual satisfaction as straight couples who are having more frequent sex*
- *More variety of sexual behaviors, including oral sex and using sex toys*
- *Longer duration of sex*
- *More orgasms and more gentle kissing*

They're also more likely to say, "I love you."[4]

When you look beyond frequency, generally speaking, lesbians have better sex than straight couples. They're more likely to have orgasms, sex lasts longer—like twice as long—and they're generally more satisfied.[5] Why? Because when they don't worry about patriarchal, penis-centric models of sexuality, they can love their sexuality as it is, without judging themselves against an irrelevant standard.[6]

"Does that sound like 'bed death' to you?" I concluded. "Saying 'I love you' through a kiss while you press a vibrator against your partner's genitals, watching her come, as you've watched her come, and she has watched you, for the last umpteen years?"

Ama and Di were silent, but their eyes said, Nope.

I continued, changing mental slides to the patriarchy of it all:

"The idea of sexual frequency as the measure of 'bed death' exists only because of the sex imperatives—the cisheteropatriarchal standards, set by cisgender men, on everyone. It fails to account for duration of sex, pleasure, connection, orgasm, or even basic satisfaction. It ignores everything that happens outside sexytimes, erasing all the moments of eroticism, connection, pleasure, and affection

throughout the day. In short, it's a problem that exists only when you accept the sex imperatives.

"So if your frequency of sexytimes has dropped, before you label it 'bed death,' notice how much aliveness does exist. If you weren't judging your frequency against some fictional standard of how often is 'often enough,' how satisfied would you be with the quality of your erotic connection? And if you want to increase the erotic aliveness in your relationship, what, apart from frequency, would increase that aliveness?"

(Even if you're not a lesbian, I encourage you to ask yourself these same questions.)

Ama tapped Di on the arm. "See? She's right. We already know teasing and play. And we already have buckets of orgasms. The main thing that's missing is just time, and Emily cannot get us more of that."

"I'm sure there are scientists working on it, but no," I said.

They fed me dessert as a thank-you for the science.

The next time I saw Di, I discovered I had sparked her curiosity; she came to me with a history lesson. Here's what she taught me:

The term "lesbian bed death" was not borne of a misogynist patriarchal narrative. It originated in the early 1980s, toward the end of the feminist "sex wars," a conflict among second-wave feminists who came to be identified as either "anti-porn" or "sex positive."

Di said, "This is a big part of the origin of the 2020s tension between trans-inclusive feminists and the other people, the ones who believe that cisgender women's comfort and convenience matter more than the safety and lives of transgender women and that trans men . . . aren't.[7]

"But!" she continued. "The good part is that in the sex-positive or 'pro-sex' rhetoric, 'lesbian bed death' referred not merely to low or no frequency of sex in lesbian relationships, but to the shrinkage of social space for public and communal discussion of sexuality within the women's movement."[8]

Her voice took on the lyrical quality I associate with her explaining her master's thesis. "As a description of a historical moment, this term resonates not as the death knell of frequent sex between lesbian partners, but as the toll of puritanical, patriarchal sex norms on women's pursuit of shared embodied liberation.

"In short, the idea of 'lesbian bed death,' as the term is used in the early twenty-first century, is yet another way to dismiss women's sexuality as inferior to men's. I'm surprised I fell for that misogynist, binary trash. But empirically and historically, I now know better and I will do better."

"I love that," I told her. "Can we keep the idea that women and femmes of all varieties deserve public and communal shame-free, judgment-free discussion of sexuality that centers their experiences, without reference to cisheteropatriarchal standards?" (And yeah, I really do talk like that in real life. But so does Di!)

She raised her water glass. "Long may we center, value, and learn from the erotic and sexual lives of women and femmes who enjoy sex with each other."

Confidence is knowing what's true, and joy is loving what's true. With a deeper understanding of both the science and the cultural history, Ama and Di understood not only how *to center pleasure, but* why *centering pleasure is part of how they make the world a better place. Their pleasure means something powerful in a world that still—still! how can it be?—still tries to legislate LGBTQIA2+ people out of public life.[9]*

The Pretty Imperatives

In the same way I wish I could write a sex advice book without talking about trauma, I wish I could write a book without addressing body image. But here we are, talking once more about the Bikini Industrial Complex, or BIC. That's my sister's name for the giant, corporate money machine that profits from your self-loathing, so it lies to you to make sure you believe that you are not merely unlovely and unlovable, but also unhealthy and immoral—slothful and greedy—if your body doesn't conform to the "ideal body" it says you should have.

As an imperative, to go along with the sex imperatives and the desire imperative, I think of it as "the pretty imperative."

The reality is your body is lovable right now, and your health can't be measured on a scale.[10] You were lied to. And the changes we experience with age are the fascinating prize we win for being lucky enough to grow older.

Black readers literally do not need me to tell them this. As Tracie Gilbert wrote in her book, *Black and Sexy: A Framework of Racialized Sexuality*, many African Americans

> *appeared well aware of the expectations presented by mainstream society to reject black femininity and black beauty, choosing instead to value them anyway. And in their own way this particular act of resistance—choosing one's self when there is no external incentive to do so—serves as a source and mechanism of sexiness development in and of itself.*

In a way, the BIC is mostly an *external* negative influence for marginalized people, while it's more of an *internal* negative influence for white people, able-bodied people, thin people, and others who seem to be so tantalizingly close to meeting the ideal that they can't help believing that goal is attainable. People of color, along with visibly disabled people, people of size, and other marginalized folks already know they will never meet the BIC's standard for the aesthetic ideal. But the closer you are, the more hope you have that maybe one day you could be beautiful enough to deserve to be treated as a complete human. The closer you are, the less likely you may be to believe me when I say your body doesn't have to be perfect to be lovable.

But let's get right to some solutions:

First, can you simply be curious about your body?

Body image issues are RAGE toward your own body—an urge to destroy. Obviously the urge to make your body not exist isn't compatible with the urge to experience erotic delights. Another space from which we might relate to our bodies is FEAR—turning away from them, avoiding, pretending they don't exist.

In *Come as You Are*, I recommend a practical way to experiment with shifting from RAGE or FEAR to SEEKING. In the "mirror exercise," you stand naked in front of a mirror, look at what you see there, and write down everything you see *that you like*. Do this over and over again, and gradually you build up immunity against the Bikini Industrial Complex. You learn over and over that you are already deserving of joy and love and kindness, because there is nothing your body can do to disqualify it from those pleasures.

In other words, *Hello, body. I literally see you. I love you. I want to know you.*

In *Burnout*, Amelia and I recommend "mess acceptance," recognizing that we can work hard to embrace our bodies exactly as they are, while the BIC continues to punish us for daring to try to love ourselves.

Hello, mess. I see you. I love you. I want to know you.

I want you to know you are allowed to like your body. And I know a lot of us struggle with that every day. We will always be working to love ourselves, in the midst of a culture that tells us not to. So I also want you to know that it's enough just to turn, with calm, warm curiosity, toward your body and toward the critical messages you've internalized.

Turning toward your own body with neutral to warm curiosity may mean turning away from those who would encourage you to conform to an ideal rather than embrace yourself as you are. As the child of immigrants, trauma therapist Sonalee Rashatwar's experience with a fatphobic culture included pressure from their parents to lose weight, even to have weight loss surgery, a pressure "rooted in love and a desire to assimilate." So often, the pressure to change our bodies to match the cultural ideal grows out of our love for others, our desire to please them, and out of their desire for us to be safe from the very real and very dangerous stigma against bodies that violate the cultural standard.

As they wrote in 2020:

> *In the body image workshops I run as a trauma therapist, I teach the concept of understanding our bodies as heirlooms. If we think about the purpose of an heirloom, it's a symbolic representation of resilience.*
>
> *We do not criticize an heirloom. We do not devalue it for its flaws and imperfections. We see heirlooms as tangible evidence of the existence of our ancestors.*
>
> *I want fat folks of color to see our bodies as essential and necessary in the context of survival. I want us to remember to write ourselves into existence at the expense of diet culture and fatphobia.*[11]

Hello, heirloom. I see you. I love you. I want to know you.

In Japanese culture, *wabi sabi* is a way of knowing the world that embraces impermanence, incorporating "flaws" and signs of age or wear into the perception of beauty. The widely discussed African ethic of *ubuntu* is generally translated into English as "I am, because we are." It locates beauty not within an individual but within community, within relationship.[12] Neither *wabi sabi* nor *ubuntu* exists to understand the beauty of our bodies, but both create a potential context for understanding bodies—our own and others'—more humanely and compassionately than the context of the BIC.

I don't think it's a coincidence that language that makes space for beauty beyond the Bikini Industrial Complex is found only in cultures outside my own white American culture. The closest I can find to a Western conception of beauty beyond the BIC is "jolie laide," a French-language term that, translated literally, means "pretty ugly." These days it's generally used to mean something like "unconventionally attractive." Unfortunately, an internet image search for the term surfaces almost exclusively photos of ultra-thin cisgender white women whose facial features are stunning but not symmetrical with mathematical precision. It highlights just how narrow is the range of "conventional" beauty.

I genuinely believe that every body is beautiful because beauty is innate in every body, just as it's innate in every flower, every bird, every rock, and every river. But I know from long experience that many more people struggle to internalize this truth than I would ever expect. If I met you, I would probably be delighted with the beauty and kindness you bring to our interaction, and then I would be stunned to realize that you, too, carry around a vicious voice in your head that tells you you don't deserve pleasure and love . . . a voice just like the one I carry around.

I'm not saying "beautiful" is something you should be; I'm saying "beautiful" is something you can't help being, because all bodies are already beautiful. Period. Human beauty isn't the same thing as the culturally constructed, aspirational aesthetic ideal. Human beauty is having any human body.

An Antidote to the Imperatives: Blanket Permission

Since I can't anticipate every single detail of what the "shoulds" or "should nots" of the sex imperatives in your garden say ought to happen during sex, let me offer blanket permission. My only rules are, as I have said, that everyone involved is glad to be there and free to leave with no unwanted consequences, and there's no unwanted pain.

You can allow a partner to ejaculate into your mouth or not, and you can choose whether to swallow or not, you and your partner can choose whether to kiss with the ejaculate between your mouths or not. You can choose to put a penis in your mouth in the first place, or not. You can use just your hands. You can use just your mouth and use your hands for something else, like touching another part of your partner's body or touching somewhere on your own body or gripping the sheets or just knitting if that's what you're into. Careful with the needles.

And if there is something you think you *should* be doing, but it hits your brakes, you do not have to do it. You can do something else, anything else. You can burst into song if you want to. You can overexplain the plot of your favorite movie. You always get to choose.

More blanket permission:

Orgasms take as long as they take, and they are only as important as you decide they are. If a person's body has a clitoris and a vagina, they're much more likely to orgasm from clitoral stimulation than vaginal stimulation, but they also might be orgasmic from many other kinds of stimulation—breast or chest stimulation, earlobe stimulation, foot stimulation, back-of-the-knee or inside-of-the-elbow stimulation, or fantasy alone, or none of these. Some people never have orgasms and never really want to, despite the pressure they feel from other people to keep trying. People vary. You are not doing it wrong. If you want to have an orgasm and haven't yet, there are books about just that (see chapter 1, endnote 2).

You also have permission to try sex toys, with or without your partner. They do not replace a partner in any way, but they can be an adjunct. When people tell me they feel threatened or intimidated or insecure around their partner's sex toy, I ask if they feel that way about their partner's car, bus, train, bicycle, or whatever mode of transport they use to get places. That vehicle does things you can't do, but you can do a whole lot of things that vehicle will never do. Try going along for the ride.

While I'm on the subject, no, you can't get addicted to a sex toy, though you can get "spoiled," in a way. For example, if you have orgasms much faster when you use a vibrator, that speed might reset your expectation about how long it "should" take to have an orgasm, which might mean that when you try to have an orgasm without the toy, maybe you begin to feel frustrated that it's "taking so long," when in fact it's just taking as long as it always takes without a vibrator. And if you start getting frustrated, is that going to make it easier to orgasm, or is it going to hit the brakes and slow you down? Right. Brakes.

Even more permission: If you want to do erotic things that do not include any genital touching, you can do that. If you want to use lube not just on the genitals but all over everyone's bodies so that everything anyone touches is slick and slippery, as long as everyone involved is glad to do that, go for it. If you want your partner to gently bite your labia, you can ask for that. If you want to thrust your tongue into your partner's ear, you can ask for that. If you want to fuck your partner's armpit and your partner is glad for you to do that, fuck your partner's armpit—it's called "axillary intercourse."

LETTING GO OF OTHER PEOPLE'S JUDGMENTS

A lot of sex books talk about letting go of fear of other people's judgments. The usual advice is to remember that people really aren't thinking about you that much! They're too absorbed in their own lives to notice the things you worry they'll judge. That is correct, and it is good advice.

But I think it ignores an important dynamic:

I've found that the people who are most worried about other people's judgments are also very busy monitoring and judging other people. Who gained weight, who didn't wear makeup to work, whose clothes aren't the right clothes? Which couple is clinging to each other at the party, which couple spent time in different social groups, which couple bickered?

If you find yourself thinking a lot about other people's appearances and behaviors and whether they're doing it "right," chances are you also think a lot about your own appearance and behaviors and whether you're doing it right. Your judgment of others and your worry about yourself are both borne of the underlying belief that there is a right way and a wrong way to be, and we are all supposed to do whatever it takes to be right, no matter how unnatural it feels, no matter how much it hurts. After all, you torture yourself to make sure your body and face and behavior are correct, and if you can (or must) do it, so can (or must) anyone and everyone else!

To let go of fear of other people's judgments of you, let go first of your judgments of yourself and others. Be who you truly are, and be compassionate toward yourself for the ways you don't match the imperatives you've been measuring yourself against. Admire others for who they truly are, especially the ways their true self doesn't match those imperatives.

You belong in the human community. You are allowed to be you, and other people are allowed to be themselves. And you'll find that as you replace your harsh self-criticism and body discipline with self-compassion and self-forgiveness, your need to judge others will evaporate, along with your fear of their judgment.

Blanket Permission for New(ish) Parents

For those who bring young, dependent humans into their lives, the imperatives become entirely implausible and have to be replaced with brand-new, wholly individual ways of experiencing erotic connection. *Of course they do.* The meanings of your individual life, your shared life, your bodies, and your identities all change, radically and permanently. Everyone who has become a parent knows this, and yet somehow many, many parents are unprepared for the truly radical changes that happen to their bodies, their relationship, and their sexual connection.

I get asked more "How am I supposed to . . . ?" questions from new parents than from anyone, and the answer is always *you are not.*

You're not supposed to do anything but your best, which is hard enough without added pressure to do what you're "supposed to."

"How am I supposed to meet the needs of my child, my employer, my partner, and all the other people in my life, and stay sane?" You are not. You are supposed to do your best, and your best will nearly always fall short of the vast, infinite sucking vortex of what the world needs from you.

"How am I supposed to feel sexy when my nipples are cracked and bleeding/I haven't slept more than three hours in a row for most of a year/I'm extremely touched-out from toddler hands on me/the sight of my partner fills me with an unfathomable rage?"

You. Are. Not.

You're not supposed to.

You know what you're supposed to do? You're supposed to collaborate with your partner to co-create a context that makes pleasure easier to access. And that is going to be very, very difficult during this time when your life is changing rapidly, continuously, and uncontrollably. It's normal for the pleasure project to drop lower on your list of priorities.

But here's what I've found, both in listening to parents talk about their struggles and in learning about their solutions:

I think you miss each other. Even when you're furious with each other, a part of you wants to find a way through all the emotion and exhaustion and existential terror, to a place of adult human connection. Parenting can be excruciatingly lonely—a bitter irony, considering one of the first things you lose when you add children to your family is *time alone*. Time with your child is many things, but it is not the same as time with a friend or time on your own, both of which are basic human needs. Finding moments to feel attuned to a fellow adult is deeply nourishing, and sexual connection is a powerful way to get that.

You want tips? I've got five for you. But none of them will help you if you use them with the goal of doing what you're "supposed to," rather than a goal of finding your way back, even if only for a few minutes, to a partner you admire and trust.

Here are your tips:

1. *Schedule a regular time to connect,* even if you don't end up having sex. You can pay attention to your emo-

tional floorplans and notice how each person can help the other get to spaces adjacent to lust, to increase the likelihood that sex might happen, but expectations and obligations mostly just hit the brakes. It helps to have a sense of humor about the struggles of finding time to be adults together while taking care of kids, but go ahead and have big fights if that's what it takes to help you clarify your needs to each other.

2. *Center pleasure.* Your shared task is to co-create a context that makes it easier to access *pleasure,* not arousal, horniness, orgasms, or desire. If you have sex you don't enjoy (maybe so you can say you had sex or cross something off the to-do list), the next time an opportunity arises, your brain will remember, "Hey, last time was no fun," and it'll be even more difficult to show up for the party.

3. *There are no rules* but consent. If one of you wants to connect sexually and the other partner is feeling exhausted but affectionate, maybe the less interested, sleep-deprived partner can be entirely lazy, lying beside their partner and watching them masturbate like they're watching TV—for fun, for amusement, for relaxation, for distraction.

4. *Overnights and weekends away,* to change the context. Narratives of parents who stay erotically connected very often include intentional time away from parenting. It's easier when, say, a family member can come stay with the kids while you get away—the context is thoroughly changed without you having to do a lot of work—but maybe it's easier if the kids spend the night with their aunt and you stay home. At home, take the first couple of hours to create a bubble of grown-up fun—in the *Come as You Are Workbook,* I call it the "Magic Circle." Decorate with lights or candles, add a gorgeous scent to the air, definitely

get all the kid toys out of the bedroom. Change the sheets, finish the dishes and the laundry, and clean the bathtub in case you want to play in the water. What an opportunity to give great choreplay! Maybe all you'll do with your time together is sleep for twelve hours, but that alone is nourishing for your bodies and your relationship.

5. Finally, when in doubt, go back to the beginning: *What is it that I want when I want sex?* What is it that I like? What activates my accelerator and what hits my brakes? Your answers are probably changing as your household, relationship, bodies, and internal experiences change. Keep talking to each other. If you can talk about another human's bodily fluids, you can talk to each other about your sex life.

Now is your moment. The old rules—the sex imperatives—never actually applied to your sex life, and the transformation that comes with adding children to your relationship is an excellent opportunity to dump all that old garbage and start from scratch. You get to play a whole new game, with a new set of rules that you invent. Precisely what the rules are and how you play by them will vary from relationship to relationship and from season to season as the tiny humans in your life grow and develop.

BONUS TIP: Your bodies are permanently different, whether you're a birthing parent or not. Don't waste time and energy trying to "get your body back"; you still have your body, it never left you. Instead, spend that time and energy learning about your body as it is now. None of the rules about how bodies "should" be ever applied to you, but now they are distracting irrelevancies that prevent you from noticing that your body is a frickin' frackin' miracle that is helping to keep other young humans alive! Your body is glorious. Care for it as you're caring for your tiny humans: Listen to your body, move it in ways that manage stress, stay connected in loving, trusting relationships with other adults, eat food that nourishes you, body and soul, and get every second of rest you can.

Another Antidote to the Sex Imperatives: Play a New Game

The rigidity and urgency of the sex imperatives set the stakes of sexual difficulties so high you might even wonder if you, your partner, or your relationship are *doomed*.

Hey, remember which space in the emotional floorplan lowers the stakes?

PLAY.

In their essay "The Pieces of the Puzzle," gender therapist Fitz offers the metaphor of sexuality as a jigsaw puzzle.[13] When you start the puzzle, they say, you begin organizing the pieces based on shape (edge or center), color, text, texture, etc., and you rely on the picture on the box to tell you what the puzzle is supposed to look like in the end. But what if the puzzle just came in a bag, with no picture to guide you? You don't even know for sure that all these pieces are from the same puzzle! Let the "unknowns" introduced by this bag of puzzle pieces spark *curiosity* rather than fear that the pieces won't fit or that you'll somehow do it "wrong."

They conclude:

> *I like to think of it as a gradual collection of puzzle pieces. Collect the ones that fit, set aside the ones that don't. Over time you'll see ways they fit together and make sense to you. You don't have to know the whole picture in order to recognize pieces you like and enjoy the experience.*

This brings me to the next antidote to the imperatives: Play a new game.

To begin, it might help to invent a name for something you want to try, like with axillary (armpit) intercourse. I've learned that people feel normalized when they find out there's a term for something. Once, after a workshop, a woman approached me and said, "I know you're going to say this is normal, but I just have to ask. What my partner really likes is when he presses the soles of his feet together and I lick into the space between his arches. Is that . . . ?"

"Sure! Totally normal," I said. I described a little about how even though our feet are pretty far from our genitals, in our brains they're right next to each other, so lots of people enjoy foot sensations. And because I have a passing familiarity with the sort of Latin roots used to invent medical terms, I added, "Let's call it 'interplantarlinctus.'" And you can try it, too, if you're interested.

Try giving a name to whatever you and your partners are curious to try. You've just given a name to the new game you're going to play together.

If you aren't sure what new game you want to play but you'd like to reveal some unspoken imperatives in your erotic mind, try a stop-start game. These kinds of games ask you to share pleasure and touch without urgency or expectation of "performance."

All you have to do is stop doing any sexual behavior at a random moment during sex and change to some other sexual behavior. Don't follow the script of what order you're supposed to go in or when you're supposed to transition to something new. If it helps you break the rules, you can make it like a game of Simon Says.

> PARTNER A: *Simon says stop sucking.*
> PARTNER B: *[stops, with a frustrated, amused grunt]*
> PARTNER A: *Simon says suck but very, very gently.*

Or,

> PARTNER A: *Stop thrusting.*
> PARTNER B: *[stops, with a frustrated, amused grunt]*
> PARTNER A: *[teasing] I didn't say "Simon says . . ."*

Not comfortable inviting Simon into your sex life? Make it Simone. Or switch to "Mother, may I?" using whatever term of endearment feels better than "Mother," like "Honey/Darling/Lover, may I?" or your partner's name. Or use "Mother"; do you!

Another game you can play? I call it "Where Lick?" Ask yourself, "What part of my partner's body have I never licked? Under what circumstances might we both be interested in the experience of me licking the unlicked part?" Talk about it. Create a sex-positive context and give it a try.

Or you might try a version of sensate focus therapy, which progresses in stages over a number of weeks. For example:

- First, Partner A touches Partner B, excluding body parts that underwear covers. Partner A's job is to touch for their own pleasure, while Partner B's job is to speak up if something feels uncomfortable. And then they switch roles.

- Next, Partner A touches Partner B, still excluding body parts that underwear covers, for *both* partners' pleasure. The "touchee" speaks up both when something feels uncomfortable and when something feels especially good. And then they switch.

- Then A touches B, *including* the body parts underwear covers, for both partners' pleasure, with all the mutual communication of the previous stage. And then they switch.

- At last, Partners A and B touch simultaneously, for mutual pleasure.

The imperatives often bubble to the surface when people explore in this more systematic way; be ready to talk about them as they emerge, either in the moment or some other time, when you're not in the middle of the experience.

Another game that can allow the imperatives to bubble up so that you can discard them is to play within the structure of the peripheral nervous system. Choose an area of your body (or a partner's) and explore it with attention to one type of sensory input at a time. Here are just a few of the different ways that human skin can experience sensations:

- Light touch—feather-soft touches that brush over the skin.

- Deep touch—pressure touch that presses down through skin to muscle below.

- Texture—try different textures, from sleek silk to rough stubble, from suede to silicone.

- Temperature—stay in a gentle range at first, of course. You're not trying to burn your partner or give them frostbite; but an ice cube moved over the surface of the skin will activate those temperature-sensitive nerve endings.

- Movement/Stillness—sensations can be fleeting, as a hand moving over and away from the surface it's stroking, or they can sustain, as a hand resting on a surface. How does touching your partner feel in your body, when you stay still and keep your touch the same for several seconds or more?

- Stretch—skin stretch, joint and muscle stretch, connective tissue stretch.

- Hair follicle displacement—can you touch your partner so lightly that you move the hairs on their body without touching their skin? Follicles have nerve endings that sense when a hair is being moved!

Don't forget what we learned in chapter 2, that our perception of a sensation varies, depending on the context. How is it with the lights on or off, at home or on vacation, in the afternoon or at midnight?

For more ideas about new games you can play, try the various card packs, dice games (like the couple in chapter 3), and books with titles like *101 Fun New Party Tricks for Sexytimes.* All make for fun inspiration, as long as you engage with them without urgency, with nothing at stake, and with no sense that there is a right or wrong way to play these games. In their book *Gender Magic,* gender and sex therapist Rae McDaniel tells the story of watching a friend, garbed in an inflatable dinosaur costume, masturbating to orgasm in front of a delighted audience at a play party.[14] You really are allowed to break every rule. It really is supposed to be fun. In chapter 2 I described pleasure as a shy animal; when you play a new game, you're crafting rules to coax the animal into a carefree romp.

The only universal rule, with all these games, is: Everyone involved is glad to be there and free to leave with no unwanted consequences. With each game you play, you collect more pieces in the puzzle of your own, your partner's, and your relationship's sexual pleasures.

If you have been reading with a sense of urgency, feeling that your relationship is at stake because of sexual difficulties, take a breath. If you've felt that the tools and mindsets from part 1 seemed impossible, take a step back. The sex imperatives have taken up residence in your emotional floorplan, and it might be time to declutter them.

No sexual difficulty is worth destroying an otherwise strong relationship. Are you showing up for each other with admiration and trust? Are you turning toward your sexuality, as it is right now, with confidence, joy, and curiosity? Then you're already doing it right, regardless of the outcome or timeline.

What's truly necessary is for you to recognize the lies you've been told and to make choices about whether to believe them or not. Do you have to follow the sex imperatives? Does your body have to be disciplined into conforming with the Bikini Industrial Complex's idea of a body worthy of pleasure? Or are you allowed to play with your partner according to whatever rules feel right for you?

You get to choose.

Chapter 9 tl;dr:

- The coital imperative, variety imperative, performance imperative, confidence imperative, pleasure imperative, relationship imperative, the desire imperative, and even the sex imperative itself—to be a sexual person who wants, has, and likes sex—could all be creating a needless sense of urgency for you to "work" on your sex life to make it more like it's "supposed" to be.

- You are already beautiful because "beautiful" is something you can't help being, just as a tree can't help being beautiful and a dog can't help it and a river can't help it. You couldn't be less than beautiful if you tried.

- To stop the impact of the sex imperatives, try playing new games by different rules that ask you to share pleasure and touch in ways that have nothing to do with any urgent need to be or do sex differently.

Some Good Questions:

- Which sex imperatives are explicitly present in my brain? Which might be implicit—unspoken yet still obstructing my access to my full erotic self?

- What would it take for me to look at my body in the mirror and see that I am already beautiful, as every tree is already beautiful in all seasons?

- What kind of game might we try to play by new rules, instead of allowing the unspoken imperatives to tell us how to live our erotic lives?

Chapter 10

THE GENDER MIRAGE

On the day you were born—or maybe even earlier—some adult looked at your genitals and declared, "It's a boy!" or "It's a girl!" or "It's an intersex child!" Along with that declaration comes a cultural "handbook"—a package of rules and regulations about how to live in this body, what kinds of toys you should play with, what kinds of people you should love, what kinds of feelings you're allowed to express and what kinds of feelings you will be punished for expressing, and lots of other obligations about what goes into being a "boy" or a "girl." Among intersex babies, the family or medical providers often pick a handbook as their best guess.[1]

This is the gender binary we hear so much about—the two social roles that we assign to people, based on their bodies. Like the sex imperatives, the gender binary is a collection of other people's opinions that we can ignore if we choose to. But the sheer tonnage of lies we've been taught about gender—our own and other people's—takes it to a whole different level from the sex imperatives. I think of it as a mirage, a shimmering optical illusion that looks so real you can't imagine that it's just a by-product of social dynamics bouncing off diverse human bodies, creating the appearance of something that isn't really there.

This mirage of rules you and your partner are supposed to follow based on the genders you were assigned are, I believe, the most pervasive and persistent barrier we face when we try to use all the tools from part 1. At the most fundamental level, if we're struggling to create change the problem isn't our partners, it isn't our changing and inconvenient bodies, it isn't even that we're stuck somewhere in our emotional floorplans, it's that we can't see our bodies, our relationships, and our world as they truly are, because we are seeing a mirage in its place. A gender mirage.

The classic mirage is water in a desert. A traveler sees an oasis in the distance, a shimmering that signals relief from the torturous aridity. But the closer the traveler gets to the mirage, the more obvious it becomes that there is no oasis. It was an optical illusion.

In our mundane, non-desert-crossing lives, such a mirage might be the shimmer of a hot roadway looking like a puddle, prompting us to drive around it.

You know how you dispel a literal mirage?

You shift your point of view. The closer you get to it, the more you see it for what it is: an illusion, created by things that were actually there but were not what your eyes told you they were.

My goal in this chapter is to facilitate enough shift in your point of view that you notice the optical illusion that is the gender binary, with its rules and regulations that have defined our lives from the day of our birth and that prevent us from seeing, understanding, and loving our bodies, our relationships, and our world as they truly are. I want to show you the illusion, describe what happens when you don't participate in the illusion, and explain how to do that. It might be my most difficult task in this book, because the mirage had decades to influence your erotic garden and you'll likely need as many decades to undo that influence. Better get started.

Before I describe the mirage in all its pleasure-adverse glory, let's make sure you've got access to the antidote: connected authenticity.

What You Need: Connected Authenticity

A classic structure for, say, a Pixar movie, is that characters start out pursuing what they want, but in the end they succeed at getting what they really *need*. What they want is the thing they believe will make them happy forever. What they need is what will *actually* make them happy forever. Mei in *Turning Red* wants to get rid of her panda, but in the end, she needs to choose to keep it. Miguel in *Coco* wants to be a musician, but what he needs is to connect to his ancestors. In *Inside Out,* Joy wants to keep Riley happy, but she needs to let Sadness call for connection ("Mom and Dad, the team," Joy realizes, "they came to help because of Sadness!").

What you want, what the gender mirage has assured you will bring you happiness, is to be an ideal "Giver," if you're a girl, or "Winner," if you're a boy (more on these soon). But what you need, what will actually bring you happiness, is to be welcomed in your community as your full, authentic self. Here's how the story goes:

Imagine a little human born into a world and given the "It's a girl!" handbook. From the very first breath, this kid is in training to be a Giver—someone who has a moral obligation to be pretty, happy, calm, generous, and unfailingly attentive to the needs of others.

An infant's life literally depends on adult caregivers meeting their needs. The surest way to get that is *to be good*, to do the things they get praised for and avoid the things they are scolded for.

So every day, our little human learns more and more about how to be a good girl. She's praised when she is pretty and happy, lavished with love when people witness her generosity and attention to the needs of others. What a good girl! Oh no, don't cry! Put a smile on that pretty face! That's right, what a sweet, pretty, nice little girl.

As she grows, she begins to experience moments when she is not a perfect Giver. She gets angry, and she is scolded for her anger. She wants something for herself, and she is called selfish. She is faster or smarter or funnier than a boy, and everyone looks away. She learns that some parts of her make her not a good girl.

No girl is the ideal Giver she is trained to be, and no girl was born to be that ideal; she is born to be her *true self*. Her true self is the gift she brings to the world, the gift she was given by God or fate or the random dice roll of the universe or whatever you believe in.

But with time, her many experiences of failing to be a good girl gradually erode her spirit, as a river carves out a canyon, until there is an unbridgeable chasm between the *ideal self* she is supposed to be and her *true self*.

But the handbook says that's not true. The handbook says a girl's gift is to be pretty, happy, calm, generous, and unfailingly attentive to the needs of others, and if she falls short, she will be punished. She *deserves* to be punished. Her skills in chemistry or languages or rugby are acceptable only insofar as they add to her being pretty, happy, calm, generous, and attentive to others' needs.

Yet even the harsh self-criticism she inflicts on herself can't drown out her inner calling to be her true self, the self she was born to be.

There will come a moment—not just once, but again and again in her life—when she will have a choice, to be a good girl or to be true to herself. To behave like an ideal Giver, or to be who she truly is.

How do you want her story to end? Do you want her to learn to behave like a perfect Giver, choosing to be a good girl and welcome in her community . . . as long as she never falls short?

Or do you want her to choose herself and be welcome in a community of people who know and love her as she truly is?

Which ending do you want for yourself?

For your daughters? For your mother?

In the best relationships, our loved ones encourage us to choose ourselves, even if it's less convenient for them.

Yet many humans spend their whole adult lives trying to be that ideal self, neglecting and disparaging their true self as unworthy of safety, love, belonging. It's a rational choice, since we want to be good enough to belong within our community. As infants, our lives literally depended on others' love and approval, and Givers are taught that our lives will always depend on it.

Boys have their own version of this split between their true selves and their ideal selves. Part of the difference between the "It's a girl!" handbook and "It's a boy!" handbook is the nature of the ideal you're told to match—not a Giver, but a Winner, strong, stoic, ambitious, independent, and infallible. Ultimately what it means to be a "good boy" *includes* "being yourself," in the face of others' objections. Indeed, boys are punished if they seem too dependent on other people's opinions and affection. The ideal of stoic individualism means that, rather than being obliged to attend to the needs of others at the expense of their own needs, boys are obliged to isolate themselves, need nothing from anyone, feel nothing more tender than loyalty or comradery.

A boy, too, like everyone, wants to be safe, held in love by his community, and to be who he was born to be. He needs authenticity in connection.

And a trans person wants the same thing, but the split between who they are and who the world tells them they should be is all the greater, and the necessity of embracing themselves as they truly are all the more urgent. They're given a handbook, just like everyone, and they do not see themselves in its pages. They hear themselves referred to by some pronoun over and over, every day, and may feel somewhere inside themselves, "Nope, that's not it," maybe not yet sure why. The world demands that they perform something incongruent with a core aspect of their true selves, yet the longing inside is the same as anyone else's: to be who they truly are, while safe within the human community.

The whole LGBTQIA2+ community, along with people of color, people of size, and disabled, neurodivergent, or chronically ill people don't need me to tell them that this is all more complex when other parts of your self, beyond your gender identity or expression, depart from the "ideal."

We all want to be safe, held in love by our community, but we need to find it without sacrificing our true selves. This is the core of "having it all"; to be free from punishment for not matching the ideal, to be loved when we are our truest selves. We need connected authenticity. This is the antidote to the gender mirage I'm about to make explicit.

Here are two conversational starting points for exploring how the "It's a girl!" and "It's a boy!" handbooks tell people to live in their bodies.[2] As you read through it, feel free to circle or highlight the parts that feel true to your personal experience, or that you feel you've noticed in a partner's experience, and draw a line through the parts that don't feel relevant.

> *An important note before we start: These are descriptions of mainstream Western culture's rules, other people's opinions about how people are supposed to live in their bodies in general and how to behave sexually in particular. They may be uncomfortable to read for anybody, even as I've tried to be playful and gentle in my approach. But for trans, nonbinary, agender, and other gender-diverse folks, these upcoming sections may read like descriptions of a violent perpetrator. I'm not trying to add that to your life. Please feel free to skim, skip ahead, or tear these pages out and ritualistically set them on fire. Do what you need to do.*

THE "IT'S A GIRL!" HANDBOOK:

5 Rules for Living in Your Body

BY
THE GENDER MIRAGE

Greetings and welcome to life! You've been assigned to the "girl" category of humanity. You're so pretty and sweet! Thanks for being so sweet!

Let's talk about some rules for living in this body.

The first rule for being a girl is that girls are the sweet, loving, attentive subordinates of boys. Weaker, nicer. We're even cleaner! We are also tough and fun and never complain that our feelings are hurt! Well, we do, but then *eye roll*, right? *Girls.* Being sweet, loving subordinates who are also tough and fun and uncomplaining is in no way contradictory!

Second rule: We adore being adored, so we will work hard to please others. We're compliant, obedient good girls who do what we're told. Being liked by boys is extremely important. Secretly it's the most important thing, even though we would never say that out loud. After all, we are also strong, independent women who don't need a man to be happy! This is in no way a contradiction.

The third rule is about emotions. Girls have a variety of emotions, but mostly we should be happy and agreeable. We're responsible for making sure everyone feels good, and if someone doesn't feel good, we make space for them to have their feelings. Their feelings—anyone's feelings, everyone's feelings—matter more than ours do, so we make sure we never inconvenience anyone with anything so troublesome as our own difficult feelings.

Sometimes we do feel sad or lonely or worried or even scared, and then we need attention, which, again, *eye roll*. We never get angry, though. Well, sometimes anger happens, but we know that it's wrong and we'll do everything we can not to let our anger make anyone uncomfortable . . . but sometimes it just builds up so much that it explodes out of us, and if people treat our anger with contempt, well . . . that's fair. That's being a girl.

Fourth rule: We are the Givers. We have a moral obligation to be pretty, happy, calm, generous, and attentive to the needs of others.[3] Because this is a moral obligation, if we ever fail to be pretty, happy, calm, generous, or attentive to the needs of others, then we have not simply failed at a task, we have failed as people. We *are* failures. And for that, we deserve to be punished. If there's no one around to punish us, we'll go ahead and beat the crap out of ourselves! We search for ways to "fix" ourselves, to be nicer, to set better boundaries, to make our bodies smaller, to love our bodies more, to be more patient, to stand up for ourselves. We sacrifice our bodies, our time and attention, our hopes and dreams, even our lives, on the altar of other people's comfort and convenience.

Which brings me to the fifth rule, the sex rule. It's very simple:

His pleasure is what matters, so be nice. It's selfish to be too insistent on experiencing pleasure yourself. Don't tell a partner what you want and like. Don't do anything to be perceived as "sexual," but also don't do anything to be perceived as "prudish." Be "great in bed," which means do everything he likes, but never draw too much attention to your sexuality. If a woman initiates sex too often, she's a slut and a whore. If she doesn't initiate often enough, she's a prude, frigid and full of sexual hang-ups. She should be easy to arouse, easy to make orgasm with vaginal penetration, easy to please.

If we wear certain clothes, go home with the guy, get drunk, or have had sex with other people, well . . . we get what we had coming. If we're not pretty enough, we're not even worth raping. Wait, what? That can't be true. Isn't that just an appalling lie someone wants us to believe because they want to decide what we should do with our bodies and think we shouldn't be allowed to—Oh, it's true? Oh. Okay.

It's true. It's um . . . it's definitely true. Our bodies aren't really ours to do with as we choose. Our bodies are in the public domain, for others to comment on, prescribe treatments for, touch, judge, have sex with, and it's our job to smile and be pleasant and try harder to have a body other people approve of and desire.

If we aren't smiling and pleased to do whatever a man wants to do, we're a bitch. If we're a lesbian, we're a man-hating bitch. If we're a feminist, we're a man-hating bitch who can't get laid. If we talk about the patriarchy, we are blaming our problems on men instead of taking responsibility for our own shortcomings; maybe if we asked more nicely, maybe if we wore different clothes or more makeup or less makeup or higher heels or lower heels or if we "waited our turn" or just worked harder or were a little more patient and supportive of the men in our lives, we'd get what we want. It's not the rules that are the problem, it's *us.* We're the problem, hi! And complaining isn't going to change that.

The emotions we're allowed to feel about all of this are: happy and occasionally sad or scared or, even more rarely, lonely. Women don't get angry and they certainly never inconvenience others with anything as ugly and uncomfortable as a difficult feeling.

These are the rules of being a girl.

Goodbye for now, and *good luck*—you're going to need it.

THE "IT'S A BOY!" HANDBOOK:

5 Rules for Living in Your Body

BY

THE GENDER MIRAGE

Greetings and welcome to life! You've been assigned to the "boy" category of humanity, which is a real honor for you—but then, it's nothing more than you deserve.

There are a few things you should know about being a boy that will help you succeed at eventually becoming a man like me. Notice how manly I am?

The first rule of being a boy is boys are better than girls. Being a boy is the opposite of being a girl and being anything remotely girly diminishes your boyness.

Second rule: Boys are big and strong in every body part—including their brains! They know everything already and have contempt for those who still are learning. A boy can tolerate any degree of pain and has contempt for those who suffer without disguise.

That brings us to the third rule: Emotions. The emotions a boy has are *anger, winning,* and *horny.* You may notice some other feelings inside you; those feelings need to *stay* inside. Sad is totally forbidden. Sad is for girls, which are the opposite of boys, so sadness diminishes your masculinity, as does its big sister, grief, and its mother, loneliness. Under specific circumstances (mostly life-and-death struggles), a boy may also be permitted to feel comradery with other men (#NoHomo), but never anything in the PANIC/GRIEF space or the FEAR space.

If you do express these emotions, you will be mocked, punished, or humiliated. That's how we help you stay on the straight and narrow. You're welcome.

Fourth rule: You Are a Winner. Winners are obliged to be

strong, stoic, ambitious, independent, and infallible. Winners have a moral obligation to fight and win, fight and win, forever. There is no win that means you can stop fighting. Fight forever.

Here's something that makes perfect sense: Boys don't need or want anything from other people, we're completely autonomous, but also we fight, win, and get laid . . . all of which require other people to participate. That makes sense.

Fifth rule: Let's talk about sex! It's extremely important.

Your worth as a man can be measured, in part, by whether and how often you put your penis in someone else's body. Therefore, when someone—particularly a girl someone—declines to allow you to put your penis in their vagina, they're not just saying, "No thanks, no penis for me right now," they're gatekeeping your worth as a man.

If you're not getting laid, you're a failure. If you wait for someone's permission before you get laid, that's you needing something from someone else, which makes you a failure. If a woman says no to you, you are a loser, which means you fail at being a Winner.

Be confident, infallible, and entitled in bed, *never* vulnerable, tender, or responsive. Remember, the first rule of being a boy is boys are better than girls, so if you're trying to have sex with a girl, the person gatekeeping your worthiness is less than you. You're letting a weak, inferior girl dominate and control you. The emotions you're allowed to have about that are angry and horny. Not lonely. Not sad.

Furthermore, the only way a boy is allowed to experience love and intimacy with a romantic partner is through sex. That's why sex is an absolutely urgent issue every day of your life. The science fact is that sex itself is not a biological drive; you will not die if you don't get it. Hunger is a drive. Thirst is a drive. Even sleep is a drive, and if you don't get that need met, you can eventually die. Sex is not one of those.[4] *But love is.* And if your only way to access this basic biological need, as essential as food and sleep, is through sex, then when someone declines to allow you to put your penis inside them, it feels like they are starving you. The stakes are life-and-death high. You *need* the sex. You need it, to be a real man, to feed your soul; you need it or else you won't exist. And the gatekeepers of sex (mostly women) are weak and meek, controllable. So you can *take* it.

Love is the one biological need for which we depend utterly on others (though, never forget, boys don't need anyone for anything) and mostly we depend on women. Fortunately, when push comes to shove, girls have a moral obligation to give you what you want, to be nice to you, to smile and be sweet, to agree warmly, and if you can't get a woman to treat you that way, you are even less than a woman.

Harsh, but you can take it. You can take any pain.

Sex is easy and predictable; your desire is constant, your erections are instantaneous, your penis is huge.[5] Men are in control of sex and of their partner. Men make women lose control; the crazier she gets, the better you are. Her loss of control, her orgasm, are measures of your worth, so make sure you make her come.

Do you feel intimidated or inadequate in the face of the sex rules? Do you ever long to abandon them in favor of connected sex that prioritizes shared pleasure without performance demand? Then you are a goddamn pussy.

Harsh, but you can take it. You can take anything.

That's it! If you have any questions—you don't have any questions. A boy already knows everything and has contempt for people who have to ask questions.

Those are the rules of being a boy.

So long, and remember: Just because you'll never win, doesn't mean you can ever stop fighting.

All of this is assigned to us based on nothing more than the shape of our genitals.

And none of it was inevitable. None of it is inherently true. None of it is really how we have to live our lives.

I want you to know what's true for you, for your partner, for your relationship, and the only way to discover that is to see yourself, your partner, and your relationship through clear eyes, without the distortions of the mirage.

No One Is Immune to the Mirage

When a friend of mine came out as lesbian in her late twenties, she was surprised to find herself in a culture that was even more rigidly "binary" than any of her heterosexual relationships had been. She told me, "It was like, you're either a butch or a femme and ne'er the twain shall meet. So many people were like, 'I have sex with you, you don't have sex with me.' And it was okay if you were a butch in the streets and a femme in the sheets, but then that's your only role in the sheets. I had more freedom in my hetero relationships than with women in that subculture."

The first time she hooked up with the partner who would become her wife and co-parent, my friend said, "Okay, every item of clothing of mine that comes off, one of yours comes off too," instead of the expectation that only the "femme" partner would be fully naked. There are plenty of people who enjoy rigid power roles in which, for example, one person is naked and the other person never is. But my friend was exploring her sexuality in a culture that said sex had to be one specific way, and the roles were "gendered," not according to people's genitals, but according to people's social presentation of gender. She was battling patriarchal expectations of rigid roles, including femme passivity and submission. But my friend was confident in herself, and she felt there were zero stakes involved in what both of them assumed was just a one-time thing.

"I had nothing to lose," she told me, "So I could be clear about who I am and what I want and what I don't want." And what she didn't want was to be locked out of any sexual engagement that gave her and her partner pleasure.

Any combination of people, of any gender identities, can find themselves stuck in the habits of the mirage. Every one of us struggles—in different ways and to different extents—to eradicate it from our gardens, including people who didn't grow up to be straight, cisgender, monogamous, and/or vanilla. But when you and your partner tend your shared erotic garden together, one of your mutual tasks is pulling the weeds of the unwanted, uninvited cultural and familial messages that pop up over and over.

It's Not Even a Binary

If you weren't raised in the white Western world, you might have been raised in a culture with a different number of gender roles. Traditional Samoan culture has three but also four.[6] These things are complicated and don't map neatly onto Western, white binary concepts. Traditional Navajo culture has four (or five—again, these things really don't translate).[7] Traditional Bugis culture, in Indonesia, has five gender categories, including gender transcendent, androgynous shamans.[8] Pre-colonial Yorùbá culture had people with different reproductive roles, of course, but no distinctions of gender.[9] None of these cultures has a "right" or "wrong" number of gender categories; there is no "ideal" or "correct" number. But they don't have two.

When I hear people insisting that humans have two genders and only two genders ("Because: biology!" they may say*), I hear them saying that Samoan people, Navajo people, and Bugis people, among so many others, are less correctly human than they are.[10]

I feel confident you don't think that. Right? Right.

So now we have two different ways of recognizing that gender is not binary: We know intersex people exist, so we know anatomical sex isn't binary, and in many cultures, social gender isn't binary. We begin to see the mirage for the illusion it is.

But without that information, binary gender—"It's a girl!" and "It's a boy!"—is so convincing! Just like the mirage of water shim-

---

* If you're thinking, "But surely, Emily, *biologically* . . . there *are* two," please see Appendix 2.

mering on the surface of a road, we are seeing something real when we see the gender binary, we're just not seeing what's actually there. What's actually there is intersex people and communities around the globe and throughout history where people with what we would call "transgender" identities are a part of daily life. It's not just two, no matter how convincing the mirage.

I don't mean that your own gender identity—the real, lived experience you have in your body, heart, and mind—is a mirage. I mean that when we assign binary gender roles to babies based on the shapes of their genitals, we're assigning them to a mirage, an illusion, not something that exists as a literal, real, universal characteristic of humans.

People who are certain the mirage is real have often invested so much time, energy, emotion, and even money in conforming with standard ideas about their assigned gender that they resent the idea that none of that was truly necessary, that they could have chosen to participate in gender in a different, more authentic-feeling way.[11]

We think it's real, we can see it, it looks so real . . . but the closer we get to it, the more obvious it becomes that it isn't really there. There are no rules we have to follow. We can be women, in whatever way feels right to us. We can be men, in whatever way feels right to us. We can be agender, in whatever way feels right to us. We can be trans, nonbinary, gender-fluid. We can wear lipstick and a three-piece suit. We can wear a silk teddy and a beard. We can love and be loved, we can fuck and be fucked, all of us. The gender mirage is just somebody else's opinion about how to live in your body. You never asked for their opinion, and you have no obligation to agree.

"BUT *HOW*, EMILY?"

I'm always looking for practices, exercise, behaviors people can implement to put new knowledge to work in their sex lives, to offer tips about *how* to implement this different understanding of what sex in a long-term relationship looks like and what obstacles we face in staying connected with someone over many years. But when it comes to the gender mirage, a lot of the work happens all by itself, while you're living your life. Like soaking a burnt pan overnight. Like planting a seed. You don't get a clean pan or a thriving seedling by doing a worksheet or even through a daily practice. You simply allow time to pass, in a supportive context. A soaking pan needs soap and water. A seedling needs just enough warmth and moisture. Liberation from the gender mirage needs trusting relationships around you and the ability to turn—oh god, not again—turn with calm, warm curiosity toward your difficult feelings.

As I said at the start of the chapter, my goal is to shift your perspective enough for the mirage to flicker, so that you can see your body, your relationships, and the world as they truly are, in all their wildness. You will have feelings about it; the truth, as we know, will set you free, but first it will piss you off. Another way I say it is: Sometimes, the path to peace goes through rage.

When people ask me how to use their awareness of the gender mirage to change their sexual connections, often they're really asking, "What do I do with all this hurt?"

You know—or you're learning—how to move through the tunnel of all the emotions you may experience as you recognize what's true and what you truly need. Allow all of it. A lot of the "how" is: Let time pass, in a positive context. Good things come.

You don't have to be in a hurry, you don't have to work hard. Let it sit. Let it soak into your mind and loosen the caked layers of lies and moral imperatives and shame.

It doesn't happen all at once, which might make you want to get in there and do something with it. But just allow yourself gradually to see the world, your relationship, your partner, and yourself differently. Talk about what you see. Grieve for the ideal selves you and your partner will never be and for the selves you might have been if you hadn't been lied to. Embrace with confidence and joy the selves you are, truly, as the shell of the mirage dissolves and you see each other fully, maybe for the first time.

How do you get what you need in your relationship, to mirage-proof it? How do you get to connected authenticity?

Admiration. Trust. Curiosity. All the skills you've learned, applied intentionally and explicitly to the ways the gender mirage intrudes on your relationship and your sexual connection.

Though most everyone I've talked to has agreed that connected authenticity is at least a good idea, some people—maybe you?—are so fearful of being alone that they absolutely would trade their true selves for certainty that a partner will never leave. They're frantically clinging to their habitual role because they've been told all their lives that that is how they earn the safety of the community's acceptance.

If you or a partner are in that place, it has probably been pretty weird to read a sex-advice-type book that doesn't provide a standard against which to measure whether you're doing it "right." The reality is, there is no ideal self to aim for. There's just you, as you are. You are already everything you need to be. And all the feelings you have about that? Turn toward them with calm, warm curiosity.

Oh yay. Another opportunity to grow as a person.

The good news is, we can be both safe *and* loved for who we are, dark struggles included. But we can't have it alone. By definition we need other people—at minimum, we need one special someone—who know our true selves and love all of us.

We get there by collaborating to mirage-proof our relationship, so that we never again let someone else's rules control how we feel about ourselves or our partner. We stay in the wisdom that everyone wants to be who they are, and they also want to be welcomed in their community, satisfying others' needs.

You can have that, when you practice being more and more who you truly are and being loved in your relationship, and knowing more and more of who your partner truly is and love them in your relationship. That's mirage-proofing.

Margot and Henry

When I tell stories like Margot and Henry's, women often say, "Well, Henry is pretty exceptional, and Margot is really lucky. Most men would get defensive; most men wouldn't just step up like that; most men . . ." So I'm going to close Margot and Henry's story by going back to the beginning. They confronted the gender mirage together early in their relationship.

Henry didn't slide into adulthood already awake to masculine privilege and the gender mirage. He came of age in the 1970s, a difficult time to know what it meant to be a good man. He screwed up a lot in the early years of his sexual relationships, and he still makes mistakes.

For example, early in their relationship Margot requested an evening centered entirely around her own pleasure, without her having to reciprocate, and Henry agreed. He loved her pleasure. The next night they spent together could be all about him. "Your pleasure is gift enough," Henry assured her.

They had a delightful experience. Margot asked for and received a long, deep, full-body massage with scented oils, followed by a long, slow make-out session, with zero expectation that she put on a show for him or give anything in return.

But then. When Margot was fully satisfied and ready to rest, Henry asked for a little more. Just a little. He asked very nicely. He pouted playfully. Could he make her come just once?

Margot felt like she had three options from which to

choose. She could just go ahead and let him do more, even though it was not what they had agreed to and it would ruin the specialness of the evening. Or she could have a good old-fashioned conniption, lashing out at him for trying to turn their evening together into something that didn't center her pleasure at all, just put hers first and then expected her to meet his expectations, like her pleasure was a transaction—she could have pleasure on her terms, but then she would have to pay for it. A tempting option. But she chose her third option.

She sighed at the ceiling in frustration and said, "You could. Of course you could. You have, often, and I've enjoyed it. But then tonight would change from the extraordinary evening we had planned, where I had a rare experience of pleasure free from obligation to do anything for a partner, into a very ordinary, typical, dare I say normal experience, where I got to feel pleasure, that's great, but then I feel guilty about it and agree to do what you want to do because apparently there is no version of the world where I can experience all the unconditional pleasure I want, no more, no less. So I figure I'll let you decide what you want this night to be. Is it the night when I learn that unconditional pleasure is possible and that I might even deserve it? Or is it just another night when I feel like your expectations are my responsibility, even when you tell me ahead of time that they aren't?"

The evening lost the sparkle it had had, so Margot decided if she couldn't have the sparkle of unconditional pleasure, she would make her point clear to him, or else she would need to redefine their relationship.

Henry said things like "I just want to feel closer to you!" and "Renegotiation is always part of our connection," and "It's not like I did something you didn't want me to do; I just asked and you were free to say no."

Margot said things like "Tell me why your desire for closeness matters more than my desire for unconditional pleasure," and "We negotiate ahead of time so that neither of us has to risk asking and being told no or being asked and having to say no."

Eventually she said, "I hate to put it this way, but whose side of this disagreement would your father be on?"

"Ah shit," Henry said.

"To your credit, he wouldn't have cared about his partner's pleasure, right? But he would definitely feel entitled to whatever he wanted, regardless of what his partner wanted. The fact that you want my pleasure doesn't make it less entitled."

Henry scrubbed his hands over his face. "Yeah."

This isn't an approach to this conversation that would work for just anyone, but Margot knew Henry genuinely hated the idea of being the same kind of man his father was: entitled, aggrieved, controlling, and deliberately cruel. "What would your father do?" was a reality check that brought Henry's gender mirage to the surface, like using a warm compress to bring a cyst to a head so that it could drain on its own.

He never begged or pouted for anything after that, except in mutually agreed upon role-play. And the next night they got to spend together, Margot did indeed invest the whole evening in his pleasure. In his younger years, Henry would probably have ejaculated multiple times during such an experience; instead, he experienced multiple full-body, ejaculation-free orgasms that left his erection intact (though at half mast, which was typical for his erections at that age) and his whole body shuddering. That's just a further benefit of rejecting the gender mirage: Sex in the context of aging, free of the hang-ups around erection, ejaculation, dominance, "making" a partner orgasm, having total control but making a partner lose control, and the other bogus performance standards that distract Winners from their own pleasure and their connection with their partner.

Seeing through the gender mirage is a lifelong project, but the rewards are so great, Henry keeps working on it.

And it's not just that he has better sex—though it is definitely that he has better sex. It's that he can continue to explore and deepen his experience of eroticism, with a spirit of adventure, play, surprises, and love.

Mirage-Proof Now, Have Better Sex for Decades

Regardless of your gender or your partners', your sexual orientation or your partners', or your generation, you grew up with weeds about boys and girls, and those weeds shape your erotic garden—both how you show up in bed and how you expect your partner to show up.

But the rejection of the gender mirage is especially crucial as human bodies age. Genitals behave differently, and because the gender handbooks are inherently ageist and ableist, aging people can no longer rely on our bodies to do what a body is "supposed" to do. If we cling to the belief that the behavior of our genitals is some kind of measure of our identity or our worth, then these predictable, ordinary age-related changes can lead to devastation of a person's self-worth or of the relationship—all because a penis doesn't get erect as reliably or arousal is more gradual or intercourse isn't as available.

So sex therapists actively recommend rejecting rigid gender roles. For example, in their book *Couple Sexuality after 60: Intimate, Pleasurable, and Satisfying,* authors Barry and Emily McCarthy (themselves in their seventies and married to each other more than fifty years) emphasize the power of what they call "female-male sexuality equity," which releases partners from gendered mandates like the intercourse imperative, in order to create space for variable, flexible sexual connections that center sensuality and playfulness. The greatest downside couples experience with this freedom from gender roles, they write, is "regret and resentment that you did not adopt the equity model earlier."[12]

LGBTQIA2+ couples, too, can benefit in their senior years from their early rejection of rigid gender roles. In *The Stonewall Genera-*

tion, Jane Fleishman highlights two aspects of sexuality that I think we can all learn from:

First, one of the most important factors associated with sexual satisfaction in LGBTQIA2+ boomers was *low internalized homophobia*—that is, that voice in your head that repeats all the worst things your culture tried to tell you about who you are. Homophobia is a central feature of the Western gender binary mirage, and these elders grew up more closeted than the generations that followed, with laws against loving who they love and medical diagnoses applied to their identities. How remarkable that they've shed those messages to embrace their sexuality as it is. No surprise it's linked to greater sexual satisfaction.

And second, the LGBTQIA2+ older adults with higher sexual satisfaction felt good in their skins. They were not as polluted by body ideals as straight older adults, perhaps because they never matched it. "I never looked good in a dress," one butch lesbian elder told Jane. Aging couldn't take away her comfort in her body, because she had already accepted so much of herself.

In short, LGBTQIA2+ elders had better sex when they rejected the gender mirage. Straight elders, too.

You can, too.

Author and sex therapist Lucie Fielding uses this charming, gentle metaphor to explain how we can embrace the extraordinary diversity of human experience:

> *Imagine you walk into an ice cream shop where there are dozens of flavors of ice cream in the case in front of you. But you look up at the menu and it just says, "Chocolate or Vanilla."*
>
> *So you choose your chocolate or your vanilla ice cream, you walk out of the shop . . . and the sidewalk is crowded with people eating rocky road or mint chocolate chip or peanut butter swirl or strawberry short cake ice cream.*
>
> *If you assumed you had to order off the menu, rather than ordering based on all the many options you could see in the case, maybe part of you is angry at the people who didn't*

*question whether or not they were allowed to order any fla-
vor, who didn't wait for permission, didn't attempt to follow an unwritten rule.*

*But what if we all assumed we could have exactly what
appealed to us, without having to limit our sense of the possible to somebody else's rules about how to choose?*

In my opinion, it's strange that so few sex advice books talk about
mirage-proofing your relationship. Every qualified expert I've read
or spoken to agrees that an essential step in experiencing sexual satisfaction throughout your whole lifetime is to work on breaking free
of the "It's a girl!" or "It's a boy!" package of rules you were assigned the day you were born. Working to follow those rules and
regulations has mostly obstructed your access to sexual pleasure, and
liberating yourself from them will expand your access to pleasure.

What if you were free to choose whatever was right for you, and
you would still fully belong within your human community? I want
us never to limit our sense of what's possible for our sexualities, never
force ourselves to conform to somebody else's opinions about our
sexualities and our bodies, always to ask ourselves and our partners,
"What's true for you? What's true for me? What's true for us?"

Chapter 10 tl;dr:

- The easily proven reality is that gender is not binary—
  the mere existence of trans, nonbinary, agender, and
  gender-fluid folks is all the evidence needed to prove
  this, but it can also help to dispel the mirage to recognize that many other cultures do not construct gender
  as a binary. Cultures can have anything from zero to
  five or more genders, and they're all as real as a culture with two genders.

- Messages about gender are ubiquitous and feel intensely urgent, but, in reality, the more we allow our-

selves to be who we truly are, without reference to who we're taught we "should" be, the freer we are to build a sense of belonging that includes our authentic selves.

- The "It's a girl!" handbook of rules for how to live in your body says you should be a Giver who happily, smilingly sacrifices your time, attention, affection, sometimes your body, your health, and even your life on the altar of other people's comfort and convenience. The "It's a boy!" handbook of rules for how to live in your body says you should be a Winner who fights and wins and fucks and needs nothing from anyone, ever.

- When we actively work to dispel the mirage, we can find what we truly need—that is, we can be safe and loved in a human community, even as our full, true selves, the selves we were born to be.

Some Good Questions:

- What rules was I taught about which emotions are acceptable in me and which are unacceptable? What do I do when I feel an unacceptable emotion? What do I do when my partner expresses an emotion that I was taught is unacceptable in them?

- When do I work to ensure that my internal experience or needs do not inconvenience or disturb my partner? How does it feel to turn toward my partner's difficult feelings with calm, warm curiosity?

- Who exactly does the world say I should be? Who exactly was I born to be? In what ways can my partner and I collaborate to create space for the true selves we were each born to be, dispelling the gender mirage to reveal ourselves as we are?

Chapter 11

HETEROSEXUAL-TYPE RELATIONSHIPS

Here in the twenty-first century, the statistical reality is that the majority of people who read this will be cisgender and either in or hoping to be in heterosexual-type relationships, and there are some extra issues these folks face that are specific to their relationships' heterosexuality. Readers in LGBTQIA2+ relationships might enjoy this chapter and even find it helpful, but this is the one part of the book that assumes the reader is cisgender and in a heterosexual-type relationship (though they may or may not identify as heterosexual). See you in chapter 12, everybody else! Straight and straight-privileged people, let's do this!*

* Straight-privileged people are folks in heterosexual-looking relationships, regardless of how either partner identifies. If your relationship looks straight enough to the world, you'll benefit from straight privileges like bringing your partner to a work function without risking gender-based discrimination or going to see your partner in the hospital and not having a biased medical provider question whether you belong

Let's start by acknowledging that everyone is in a different place in terms of their relationship to the gender mirage's handbooks. My own dude came partially pre-mirage-proofed by a family full of sisters, a strong mother, and a kind of neurodivergence that meant he couldn't relate to the boys he went to school with. Other dudes . . . this is going to sound egregious, but it's true: Some dudes go to their wives' oncology appointments, listen to the side effects of radiation or chemotherapy, and say, "But she'll still be able to cook, right?"

Women, too, are in different places in their movement away from the mirage. I never felt my role as a Giver very strongly, partly because of my own neurodivergence and partly because my family of origin was so misogynist that I learned not to associate myself with anything feminine, to avoid my father's contempt. Other women . . . well, for example, my sister led a Burnout workshop with a group of C-suite executive women, and one of them asked how to stop checking her email in the middle of the night.

Amelia said, "Would it surprise you to learn that there are people who wouldn't even consider answering their email until nine A.M.?"

And the high-achieving, brilliant, feminist C-suite exec said, "That had never occurred to me."

We're all in different places. But we can all benefit from looking more closely at the gender mirage and considering the ways it might be interfering with our erotic life.

When You Keep Having the Same Fight, Maybe It's the Mirage

If you or your partner are stuck in resentment or frustration or normal marital hatred or any of the pleasure-adverse spaces, this section is for you. Similarly, if you keep having the same arguments

---

there, etc. It feels gross to be treated well because you "look straight," and all the while your queer heart is raging. Nevertheless, your cisgender, heterosexual-type relationship may be affected by the habits of the gender mirage.

about sex (or anything else) over and over again, this section will be important. If you've tried a lot of what's in this book and are still stuck and struggling, unhappy and full of complaints, this section is about the mindset shift that will get you unstuck.

To explain it, I want to talk about an asymmetry at the core of men's and women's complaints about each other. To illustrate, here's a nonexhaustive list of some of the most common complaints husbands and wives have about each other.[1]

WOMEN COMPLAIN THAT MEN:

- Don't know basic life skills like cooking the simplest meal.

- Don't even do simple things like picking up after themselves, without being nagged—"I would love to stop nagging, but it's literally the only way he contributes *at all.*"

- Just want sex and don't want to be *intimate.*

- Are always out doing their own thing instead of being with the family.

- Don't appreciate the women in their lives or the many ways women make their lives better.

MEN COMPLAIN THAT WOMEN:

- Are always complaining and criticizing; a guy can't do anything right—not parenting, not doing the dishes, not even having a basic conversation. "If she's just going to criticize me, why bother trying?"

- Are not interested in sex, or are too interested in sex.

- Try to control everything and they overreact when they don't get what they want.

- Prioritize the kids over their spouses; they have no life, nothing interesting that they do away from the family or work.

- Don't appreciate the men in their lives or the ways men make their lives better.

Do you see it? The asymmetry?

Women complain about men following the Winner rules. Men complain about women *not* following the Giver rules.

Why the asymmetry? Simple. The rules themselves are asymmetrical, rigged in Winners' favor. Givers are trying to dig themselves out from under centuries and millennia of being morally obligated to prioritize everyone else's comfort and convenience over their own. Winners, meanwhile, feel like they could lose everything if both they and their Giver partner don't follow the rules.

But far bigger than the asymmetry is the universal characteristic of all these complaints: Above all, *everyone* feels underappreciated. Everyone feels under-loved. At the bottom of all these complaints is an enduring ache of longing. "You don't love me enough. Love me more. Just love me."

The core problem is that the rules—following the rules, breaking the rules, the mere existence of the rules—are obstructing people's access to expressing and receiving love.

Women to men: Stop following those terrible rules so you can love me!

Men to women: Follow your rules so you can love me!

There is a solution! It will be familiar to readers who have also read *Burnout:*

Remember who the real enemy is.

In the Hunger Games series, Katniss Everdeen is about to enter a "game" where only one person will come out alive, so she needs to fight for her life, which could mean killing others. The whole thing is broadcast like reality TV.

Her mentor gives her this advice: "Remember who the real enemy is."

Her enemies are not the other people trapped in the deadly game with her; the real enemy is the game itself and the system that trapped them there. And you win by *refusing to play by their rules.*

When Katniss is in the game, being hunted by other players and not knowing whom she can trust, she turns her bow and arrow on a guy who might mean her no harm or might want to kill her.

He says, "Remember who the real enemy is."

Recognizing that he is not there to harm her, Katniss raises her bow and arrow to the sky—to the dome that encloses the game. She shoots her arrow at the real enemy, the game itself.

When you are stuck in pleasure-adverse spaces, full of complaints and struggling to trust and admire your partner, or if they feel that way about you, your partner is not the enemy. Your complaints are not ultimately about them; your complaints are about the system that trapped you together in this bogus game where nobody wins. It is the gender mirage's rules, far more often than an individual's personal failings, that stand between you and feeling fully, joyfully loved.

In arguments where the real enemy is the gender mirage and not your partner, either a woman appears to be failing to live up to the gendered expectations set by the gender mirage, or a man appears to be living down to the expectations women have been trained to expect from men. It might look like these kinds of conflicts:

- Small things like "my partner doesn't wipe down the shower walls after they take a shower" or "they leave a mug in the sink right after I did all the dishes" feels personal, disrespectful, or like "therefore *they do not love me!*"

- Disagreements turn into power struggles about who's "right" and who's "wrong" or who gets their way and who has to surrender.

- Your strategy to win an argument is either to harangue your partner until they give up or to stonewall them until they shut up.

- Fights include phrases like "You're just like your father!" or "You're even worse than your mother!"

- You've seen your conflict on a sitcom.

- A question could be answered with a quick internet search, yet you argue instead of looking it up.

- You can't find a way to have a sense of humor about the ordinary life issues that activate such big emotions.

- Above all, you keep having the same fight over and over, without making any progress.

These kinds of disagreements, arguments, and fights would not exist if it weren't for the gender mirage. It has trapped you in a vicious, endless game, and it is the real enemy, not your partner. You didn't spot it, because the gender mirage is so embedded in how we see ourselves, our partners, and our relationships that it's difficult to imagine what we, our partners, and our relationships would be like without it.

Redirect your anger, resentment, frustration, and hatred away from your partner and toward your mutual enemy: the collection of harmful lies that are interfering with your ability to see your partner for who they truly are and love them for it.

The "game" of the gender mirage is another "third thing." But this time, instead of turning toward it with joint fascination or joy, turn toward it as a mutual enemy. Your partner is your ally in this fight against the mirage of who you're each "supposed" to be. Together, you can turn toward it with a mutual longing to eradicate it from your relationship. It is the weeds in the garden, strangulating everything you want to thrive.

Notice when you're having a fight that follows the rules of the gender mirage—she wants him to quit being a Winner; he wants her to be a more perfect Giver—and turn your ire away from each other and toward the mirage. Solve the problem pragmatically, thoughtfully, and compassionately, in defiance of the gender mirage's rules.

One quick example: I got an email from a guy who had listened to the podcast my sister and I made, based on our book, *Burnout*. On the podcast, we said, "Turn toward difficult feelings with kindness and compassion," so often that we ultimately started saying, "kindness and motherfucking compassion," because in the end, we really do just have to be as nice to each other and ourselves as we can manage, but *ugh*, sometimes it is so hard. He told us he and his wife had started using the phrase during arguments. When one of them would notice they were falling into old patterns, like repeating themselves without listening, they would pause, and one would groan to the other, "Kindness and motherfucking compassion." Then they would keep fighting, feeling a little gentler with each other and themselves, as they did the slow work of liberating themselves from the gender mirage.

This is, of course, so much easier said than done, and it isn't even that easy to say. But it's the real, deep solution to overcoming the barriers that stand between you and the strong long-term sexual connection you're trying to create in a heterosexual-type relationship. It's the biggest, worst enemy standing between you and the love you long for.

It will take time and intentional effort and many imperfect attempts before you find a way to put this into action.

Good things come.

For Men

Hi, guys. I have bad news and then good news.

The bad news: Part of my process for writing this book was gathering stories from people about how they had improved their relationships. As you read earlier, couples that include people of the same gender or at least one nonbinary partner bring to their relationship a lot of self-reflection and an openness to thinking about their cultural understanding of gender, even when they also bring a bunch of the same unexamined assumptions that straight partners bring to their relationships.

But when I talked to straight people, it was a different story—and let me be honest: It was the same different story over and over again.

I ask a straight couple, "Tell me about some ways you've worked on your sexual relationship."

And the woman in the relationship says, "Well, it has been a process and I had to lose my shit a few times, but gradually he has learned not to assume he's entitled to . . . sex/care/service/convenience."

For example:

"When I realized that my responsive desire is not worse than his spontaneous desire, I finally stood my ground and was like, 'Not wanting to have sex with you does not make me broken! Maybe you're the one who needs to do a better job of helping me to create a context where I actually do want sex. Maybe instead of telling me I need to work harder on wanting sex, *you* need to work harder on making it easier for me to want it.'"

Or "When I started grad school while we were both still working full-time, he was really supportive and showed up for me and our family, and I was thanking him for that, telling him how grateful I was, and I said, 'It feels like I have a wife!' and he got angry. He was so offended! I had to point out, 'I'm a wife. What does it mean that you find it offensive to be called one?'"

Over and over, long-term straight sexual relationships were improved when a woman stood her ground and instructed her partner in how not to be a Winner.

I looked for alternative narratives. Here's the most varied response I found: "When my partner and I opened up our relationship, the other women he partnered with did a great job of pushing him to understand emotional labor and femmes."

In short, it took a village of femmes to mirage-proof a dude.

If you're an exception to this rule, I am thrilled. I'm married to one, so I know you exist! I want to throw a party for all the guys who worked out for themselves that being a Winner is a scam and a trap. I want to congratulate you on one particular characteristic I've noticed y'all have, that other guys are still developing: When your partner has a need that seems beyond your ability to meet it, instead of feeling like she's "high maintenance" or you're useless, you stretch yourself to meet the need, whether by learning a new skill, asking someone else to help, or meeting the need imperfectly.

But this section is here because, after talking to dozens of couples and many therapists and other helping professionals, it's clear that the "It's a boy!" handbook not only gives straight guys permission to wait until their partners complain before they so much as consider change, it might even punish guys for working toward freeing themselves from the scam of Winning.

Like, "What are you, a pussy?"

Like, "I don't know what's wrong with you, man; if a woman's breathing, I'm ready to go."

Like, "Are you gonna let her control you like that?"

It sucks.

You're trapped in a situation where your partner is asking for change and the world judges and punishes you if you change. Terrence Real wrote about it in *How Can I Get Through to You?*, saying,

> *Despite our raised consciousness and good intentions, boys today, no less than ever before, are permeated with an inescapable set of highly constricting roles. Those boys who try to step out of the box, place themselves in harm's way since, even today, our culture's tolerance for young men who deviate from what we deem "masculine" is limited and our intolerance expresses itself in emphatically ugly ways. The great bind is that those boys who do not resist, who choose or are coerced to comply, do not escape either. Avoiding attack from without, those who adopt the traditions of male stoicism and self-reliance, risk injury to the deepest and most alive aspects of their own being. The consequence of opposition is psychological and often physical brutality. The consequence of compliance is emotional truncation, numbness, and isolation.*

That means this mirage-proofing project is probably going to be more difficult for you than for your partner, because you were never allowed to learn these skills, and the other men in your life might not be able to help you develop your skills. Instead they might feel obliged to mock you if you dare to ask.

Which means you're going to ask for your partner's help to create change.

And that might seem like a bad idea, especially if it feels like she's mad at you a lot of the time. But if your partner has complained that you're not carrying your weight, or that you're not respecting her need to be a person in her own right, or that you're assuming she's there to meet your needs the way a mommy is there to meet a child's needs . . . your first assumption should be that she is offering a literal and exact description of what's happening.

Yet part of you doesn't understand why she's complaining; you're doing exactly what the world taught you to do, exactly as you have always done. She's yelling because you're being a Winner *correctly*. What's her problem?

This is the hard part, so read this sentence twice: Being a good Winner is not compatible with being a good partner.

But consider this: She is complaining because she has hope that you can become a good partner and she still feels like you are worth her effort. If she's complaining, she's trying to find a way to be with you. The least you can do is seriously consider the possibility that her complaint is entirely valid.

Does this mean she's doing nothing wrong? Of course not! But you will only be able to communicate your own complaints effectively when you learn to communicate less like a Winner and more like a good partner.

So what do you do to be a good partner? Listen to her, which Winners aren't supposed to do. Ask her what she needs, and then do it—which Winners aren't supposed to do.

Another quick reminder: If not getting sex feels like something bad is happening to you, then sex is a placeholder for something else—for love, for a sense of identity, for a feeling of success, for any of the other things you can want when you want sex. There are countless ways to get those other needs met.

But that brings me to the good news: If you want to fast-track your relationship toward strengthening your long-term erotic connection, you have that power! I did hear from a handful of straight women about the impact of being with a dude they didn't have to scold or train or argue into not being an entitled Winner. One woman told me:

> *Thankfully my last partner didn't ascribe to a lot of gendered sex ideas (he wanted me to dominate him, he wanted to give to me, he enjoyed sex of all forms and didn't think only p + v was valid). This helped me patriarchy-proof my sexuality in ways I didn't even know it needed. . . . I discovered through him that men were lovable and whole damn people with empathy. This was also because he was totally willing to show me his tenderness, too. He didn't hold back on expressing care. I fell in love with him when he put my socks on for me!*

You have the potential to be the best lover your partner has ever had and thus to have the best sex of your life. Bring to your partner questions about *her* experience and ideas for how you might change or support her or try something completely different.

I want to acknowledge that this might feel unsatisfactory to you. There might be part of you that's realizing that when you ask, "Why is this so complicated? What does she even want?" what you truly want to know is "What do I have to give her, so that she will give me what *I* want?"

It's not a trivial question, and I won't give you a trivial answer. What I'll offer is, first, the best piece of relationship advice I ever received and, second, my own dude's answer to the question.

First, when I was in my first serious relationship, my grandmother really liked my boyfriend. I was twenty, by which age every woman in every previous generation of my family had married and most had started having babies. So she gave me this advice, thinking I might be ready to use it: "When two people in a marriage give fifty-fifty, you have half a relationship. Both people need to give one hundred percent."

So for the part of you that wonders, *What do I give her, so that I will get what I want?*, the answer is: your whole self.

You're allowed to wonder what your partner wants so that you can make it easier for her to meet your wants. But never lose sight of the truth that the first priority is simply to wonder what your partner wants, regardless of whether or not it helps her meet your wants. If you show up for her freedom to be her true self, you will never make it harder for her to show up for yours.

Which brings me to my dude. He says: "Eighty percent of what's required to sustain a strong sexual connection has nothing to do with sex. Don't fight about sex, don't focus on it, focus on being in a whole relationship. Really be with each other when you're together.

"And be aware that you were scammed by masculinity. Sit with that fact and ask yourself questions about it. Maybe be mad about it, and chop some wood or whatever to purge the anger. Create some change for yourself around letting go of the lies before you ever approach your partner about it.

"The twenty percent that's about sex is the easy part. Enjoy her pleasure as much as you enjoy your own. Notice and talk about the barriers, big and small, that stand between you and the sex you like. Collaborate to get rid of those barriers. The most important difference that comes from being married to a sex educator is we can talk easily about these things without judgment or blame. It's like we're always planning for a vacation, and the more we plan, the more vacation we get."

One last tip: You will never be done learning. If you grow hugely in one relationship, that doesn't mean you're now a feminist superhero who can do no wrong. The "It's a boy!" handbook is sneaky and pervasive. You will find yourself presented with an opportunity to grow more, to integrate new insights into the way you navigate the habits of being a Winner. Your first instinct may be to fight it, like "Haven't I done enough growing and changing? Isn't this as much as my partner or even the world has any right to expect from me?" It makes total sense that it might feel that way; that's the entitlement of being a Winner. Note the habit, say to yourself, "Dang it! More Winner crap!" and choose whether to cultivate or weed.

THEY MEAN IT WHEN THEY SAY YOU'RE SEXY

A few years ago I attended a Dads Panel at a maternal health conference, and what I heard there echoed many, many conversations I've had with men over the last decade. These dads from a wide variety of backgrounds all said, "There was no time during her pregnancy or since then, when I was less attracted to my wife. She was sexy before she got pregnant, she was sexy when she was pregnant, she was sexy after she had the baby. My wife is sexy."

Are there men who find themselves not attracted to a partner whose body changes? Yeah, I've talked to those guys, too. I find that most often they view their wife's conventional beauty as a marker of their own status, as if having a wife other people want to have sex with is a sign that they're big shots. Some men are douchebags, we know this.

But the vast majority of men not only love their wives but are turned on by their bodies, through literal thick and thin. We can believe them when they say it.

For Women

There is a paradox at the heart of eliminating the gender mirage in your relationship, which is that you will have to help your dude. So I'm going to spend most of this section for you . . . talking about him. Sigh.

On the one hand, it's easy to want your partner to help more with the work of sustaining a functional household. It's easy to want your partner to be more emotionally available, more communicative, more attentive. It's easy to want him to show up erotically in a way that matches your energy. And if you've spent your life being taught that it's your job to take care of everyone else's feelings, it's easy and appealing to believe that making your relationship less binary will mean you no longer have to take care of everyone else's feelings! Sweet relief!

But on the other hand, as your dude weeds his garden, he's going to have feelings. For a lot of dudes, rejecting rigid gender roles activates an agonizing chaos of rage at the world for setting a toxic standard and punishing him for failing to achieve it, plus grief for all the moments of connection and love and joy he missed because he was busy trying to be a Winner. And, on top of the rage and grief, there's the existential despair, not knowing who he even is if he's not a Human Winner instead of a person.

So he's going to have big, difficult feelings and he's going to need your help, because the very nature of the masculinity trap he's struggling to escape means that he has not yet learned the skills to deal with those feelings, whether alone or in connection with you or anyone else.

He might say something that means "How can you still love me if I don't do masculinity the only way I was ever taught to? Who even am I?"

Or "I spent so many years trying to be one kind of man and now I see that I missed out on so much—so much love, so much connection, so much being myself. And I can never get that time back, I can never go back and get those experiences."

Or "I'm so angry about the lies I was told and the effort I wasted and how now I have to do all this extra work just to be who I am, and I don't know what to do with all this anger."

In the courageous, beautiful moment when he comes to you with difficult, vulnerable feelings that he needs help with, you may experience two uncomfortable parts of yourself. First, you may experience a part of you that slips right back into being a Giver and treats his difficult feelings as something you need to take care of. But second, you may experience a part of you that resents the hell out of being handed one more thing that's apparently your responsibility, when so much of the goal of this whole project was to get you more help, more support, more connection, more kindness and compassion, but here you are being made responsible for somebody else's shit again! That first part of you may want to take on all the labor of holding his difficult feelings for him. And that second part of you may want to reject your dude's difficult feelings, may want to push him and his feelings right back into their masculinity box where he can go deal with his own shit because you do not need another damn project. You already have more than enough to do, and he's supposed to be helping, not making more work for you. This part of you is not ready for what you find under the armor of his Winner mode.

bell hooks wrote about this in *The Will to Change,* saying, "The masculine pretense is that real men feel no pain. The reality is that men are hurting and that the whole culture responds to them by saying, 'Please do not tell us what you feel.'" bell hooks encourages women to accept the gift of a man's emotional vulnerability. Yet, we can't let men's emotions become another project women have to put on their to-do lists.

Between the two conflicted parts of yourself, there is a wise part that is aware of your decades of being a good girl, of taking care of others, a part of you that knows just how bone-tired you are of trying to be and do everything everyone expects. That wise part of you is also aware of your dude as a human who may also be bone-tired and is probably scared half out of his mind by the risk he's taking in bringing you his difficult feelings.

He may slip into wanting from you what he has always before received, the "taking care of" energy that both excuses and obstructs him from the difficult work of staying with an uncomfortable feeling until his body moves all the way through it. But in this magical moment when you truly mirage-proof your relationship, he'll experience what adults give and receive in relationships: full respect for each person's capacity to feel their feelings, without needing you to feel them for him. You will be with him as he experiences his difficult feelings, without trying to feel his feelings for him.

All you have to be is present, tuned in.

I like to think about it with this metaphor: Suppose your partner is trying to move a piece of furniture upstairs and he says, "I could use some help with this," and you, too, are trying to move your own piece of furniture upstairs. The tempting, easy answer to your partner is "I can't help you, I'm dealing with my own thing."

But the fact is you, as a partnership, need to get both pieces of furniture up the stairs. You thought it would be more efficient if you each carried one, instead of both of you carrying one at a time together, but it turns out you were wrong. The furniture was too heavy. You need to rethink your plan.

His difficult feelings are real and they are heavy, and he genuinely needs help with them. Whose job is that? His alone? That can't be, that's being a Winner, the "It's a boy!" handbook isolating a man with his difficult feelings, behind a wall of shame. But is it your job alone? No, that's being a Giver, the "It's a girl!" handbook; in reality, you do not have to carry everyone's heavy stuff.

Instead, his difficult feelings (like your difficult feelings) are a shared responsibility. Like that heavy piece of furniture, these cumbersome feelings are a third thing that you share between you. His feelings aren't him; your feelings aren't you. They exist in the space between you, pulling you toward each other or pushing you apart. Together, you turn your shared gaze toward the emotions. This is your shared project. Let it be a site of joint exploration and curiosity.

That is not the same as "Yes, I will help you with that." Maybe, to return to the furniture metaphor, his couch is well within his capacity to carry himself, but he's simply never had to carry something on his own before. In that case, your job is to stand at the bottom of the stairs, as he struggles. You can encourage and be a safety net. You can be there for him, available, responsive, and engaged, without taking on responsibility for his feelings.

If either partner says, "I could use more help with X," the correct answer, even when you're loaded with your own stuff, is "Let's see what we need to do, to get everybody's needs met."

In the delicate, beautiful, brave moment when a dude turns toward his partner with a difficult feeling, you're both standing together at the edge of your garden and he is showing the damage done by the strangulating weeds of the binary.

You already know what to do when that happens.

Hello, damage. I see you. I love you. I want to know you.

Mike and Kendra

Mike and Kendra's sex coaching petered out. Even though Mike was the one who wanted more sex, Kendra was having to remind him about their plans and make sure their home-work actually got done. She decided that if it wasn't impor-tant enough for him to follow through without her nagging him about it, then it wasn't important enough to justify nagging.

Now here they were, spending a weekend together at a sex education workshop that I was leading. They had arrived at last.

During a break on Saturday, they told me that their trouble was that he wanted, above all, to feel wanted, *as so many of us do. He told me how feeling wanted helped him to feel accepted and loved. It was nice to see he was already willing to be that vulnerable, so I had hope for them right away.*

I asked Kendra, "Do you want him?"

Sometimes when I ask a question like this, the person will hesitate and not make eye contact and I know there's some-thing deeper going on. But there was no difficult feeling here to turn toward with calm, warm curiosity. Kendra looked right at Mike and said, "Yes! You know I do. What I don't want is to feel pressured or broken or like I'm fail-ing."

More hope!

At this point, it looked like they were stuck in a classic chasing dynamic, where the more the higher-desire partner asks, the more pressured and unwilling the lower-desire partner feels, and the more the lower-desire partner says no, the more the higher-desire partner feels frustrated and re-

jected and motivated to continue asking, which makes the lower-desire partner even more unwilling . . . and so on.

I suggested what I often suggest to disrupt the chase: Take sex entirely off the table.

"For how long?" Mike asked.

I said, "Only you two know the answer to that, so I'll just throw out a time and you can start with your feelings about that." Knowing they had been dealing with this since she got pregnant with their first child, who was now preschool age, I said, "What if you tried three months?"

Mike rolled his eyes and heavy-sighed at the suggestion.

And there it was.

I'm not a therapist, but even I can recognize contempt when I see it.

Their problem was not merely that he wanted to feel wanted; it wasn't that he had an old emotional wound that felt soothed by feeling wanted; it was that, somewhere deep down, he felt like he shouldn't have to give up anything, even for a comparatively short time, to get the sex he wanted, regardless of anything he said or did. He was following Winner rules, and neither of them noticed it, because both of them believed, on some level, that he was entitled to her spontaneous desire and that she, as a Giver, was failing when it didn't happen.

The gender mirage was hiding in plain sight.

In the moment of the heavy sigh, Mike and Kendra's emotional connection vanished. They did not turn toward his difficult feeling, because they could barely bring themselves to notice it was there. They couldn't see that they both expected Kendra to carry the heavy burden of Mike's longing to be longed for.

I saw it because I was on the outside. So I asked Mike, "How do you think Kendra feels, seeing you react that way to the idea of taking sex off the table for a few months?"

"I don't know . . ." he said. He looked surprised to notice that he had had a reaction at all.

Then I asked Kendra, "How does it make you feel to see him react that way?"

She replied with a long list of feelings, and none of them was positive. Above all, she told him, "I feel like I'm a problem that has to be solved so you can be happy. Like I should just go ahead and have sex when I'm not really into it just so you don't feel deprived, but when I do that, you react this same way, you huff and look away, and what that tells me is that nothing I do is right. Not having sex with you isn't right. Agreeing to have sex with you isn't right. So I might as well not have sex with you."

I asked, "And feeling like nothing you do is right, that you're a problem to be solved, is that activating your accelerator or is that hitting your brakes?"

"Brakes! Brakes!" she said. "Because it's not even that he wants me to have sex with him, it's that he wants me to want to have sex with him, and how am I supposed to want sex with someone who thinks there's something wrong with me if I don't want to have sex with him?"

And there was as explicit a statement as I could imagine of the paradox inherent in a sexual relationship between a Winner and a Giver. Yet even as they were describing it so clearly, they weren't seeing it.

So finally I prompted, "Let's compare what's been happening to the rules of the gender mirage. Mike, I know that if I asked if you felt entitled to Kendra's spontaneous desire, you'd say no. But when we look at your choices, we can see the entitlement. For example, you've both agreed that Kendra's lack of spontaneous desire is the problem, but you could have agreed that, say, your desire for her spontaneous desire is the problem, or even, dare I suggest, you could have agreed that your mutual obedience to the desire imperatives and the gender mirage is the problem. And why are we even talking about desire and frequency, when we should be talking about pleasure? Because you're following the desire imperative and the rules of the gender mirage."

They tried again. They went back and forth until Kendra felt sure Mike understood what impact his unspoken entitlement had on her, and Mike felt sure his entitlement was not what he wanted to feel. This was the part of the conversation where I learned about her early attempts to prioritize pleasure and his shocked realization that his desire for her desire was actually a desire for her wholehearted acceptance of parts of himself that he wasn't sure were acceptable. Kendra explained why they hadn't continued with the sex coach, and I turned to Mike. "If I asked you if you felt entitled to Kendra's labor to keep the sex coaching on track, you would say no, right?"

Mike saw where I was going.

"It was invisible," he said. "In my head, her wanting to do the exercises just took the place of her wanting sex. Dang it." As he processed more, he cried (yay!), letting go of his old response to create space for a new one.

Finally I said, "Let's try again. My suggestion, for what it's worth, is to take sex off the table for several months. How do you feel about that?"

Mike's reaction was totally different. Instead of expressing contempt borne of entitlement, he looked at his hands and said to Kendra, "It feels strange . . . like, counterproductive? . . . to take sex away, when what I want is more sex. But what I really want when I want sex is for you to have the space you need to make wanting sex easy."

"Taking sex off the table will help with that," Kendra said.

"To make liking sex easy," I threw in. (The desire imperative is stubborn.)

At the end of the weekend, they found me for a moment to tell me that they had had great sex that morning. They attributed it to the new vulnerability between them. I'm inclined to attribute it to their multi-year journey toward each other, co-creating a context that made it just that little bit easier to access pleasure.

*It will take ongoing attention to keep noticing the gen-
der mirage and eradicating it from their shared erotic garden. But they have a shared language now, and, better yet,
a shared goal: Pleasure, free of other people's ideas about
what that should look like.*

The Biggest Lie

There is a foundational lie at the center of both the handbooks.
The lie is that men are simple—they're Winners who get angry or
horny—while women are so unfathomably complex, even *we* can't
understand ourselves, so how is anyone else supposed to?[2]

This lie existed before Freud, but he really put it on the map. He
reportedly said:

*The great question that has never been answered, and which
I have not yet been able to answer, despite my thirty years of
research into the feminine soul, is "What does a woman
want?"*[3]

At the same time Freud's psychoanalytic movement was building in Europe and Freud was trying to figure out what women
want, women in America were chanting their demands.

"Give us Bread, and Roses, too!"

In the fight for women's suffrage in the United States, bread was
"home, shelter, and security" and Roses were "music, education,
nature, and books." It was 1910.[4]

As a political slogan in the workers' rights movement, "bread
and roses" meant fair wages, yes, but also dignified working conditions. It meant a life not limited to bare existence, but one filled
with self-respect, "more leisure and greater freedom of action." It
was 1918.[5]

In the midst of the overwhelmingly white labor and suffrage
movements, Black women of the same era were, in the words of
professor and author Saidiya Hartman, "in open rebellion. They

struggled to create autonomous and beautiful lives, to escape the new forms of servitude awaiting them, and to live as if they were free."[6]

Autonomous and beautiful lives.

Bread and roses.

Belonging—safety in the human community—and authenticity—living as our true selves. It's what we all need. It wasn't complicated in chapter 10, and it isn't complicated now.

Freud wrote, "Women oppose change, receive passively, and add nothing of their own."[7] It was 1925.

A Freud scholar wrote, "All in all: Freud's helpless question 'What does a woman want?' . . . remains open and points to the complex character of the psychosexual development of women."[8] It was 2006.

Head-desk.

Mike and Kendra believed that Mike's desire for sex, his desire to be desired, was simple, and Kendra's lack of desire for someone who perceived her as a problem was complicated. Mike's desire was for Kendra to change so that he didn't have to, because Winners are never the problem; it's always the Giver's job to change. In reality, Kendra's lack of desire was simple: She didn't want to have sex in a context where she felt broken and obligated. Who would?

Can we agree to discard the idea that women are inexplicable and men are simple? Can we agree that, in heterosexual-type relationships, when you're stuck, it could well be because you're assuming the guy's motivations and experience are as simple as possible, and it's the woman who's got complicated problems probably stemming from her childhood? Everyone has complicated problems stemming from their childhood! All of us have been lied to.

The truth is that, though the details differ and people's access is not equal, we all need the same fundamental things. We need the freedom to be our true selves, with the safety of belonging.

Belonging and authenticity. Bread and roses. Beautiful and autonomous lives.

The question is not, and never has been, "What does my partner want?"

It is, and always has been, "How do I help them be free to be themselves?"

Chapter 11 tl;dr:

- Heterosexual-type relationships have an extra level of difficulty because the gender mirage is harder to spot in a relationship that appears so similar to the mirage.

- Dudes: Begin by assuming that your partner's complaints are accurate and entirely valid, and go from there. Then practice turning toward her difficult feelings with calm, warm curiosity.

- Women: He's going to need your help; the world really tried to prevent him from learning how to be a good partner. Don't take on responsibility for his difficult feelings, just stay with him while he learns how to tolerate them.

- The super-secret lie at the core of heterosexual-type relationships is that men are simple and women are unfathomable. In reality, we all want the same thing—to be welcome in connection, precisely as we are.

Some Good Questions:

FOR HIM:

- How does it feel to recognize that the world has refused to teach me how to be present for my partner's and even my own difficult feelings—which, it turns out, is a really important skill?

- What am I willing to do, how much am I willing to learn and grow, in order to have the sexual connection of my dreams?

FOR HER:

- How does it feel to recognize that the world probably refused to teach my partner how to be present for my difficult feelings?

- What's the worst thing that could happen if I treated everyone's difficult things in my relationship as a "third thing," a shared responsibility, not all mine and not all his? What's the best thing that could happen?

FOR ALL:

- What might it look like if we each felt fully welcome in our relationship, difficult feelings and all? How would we change as individuals and as a relationship?

- What help would we potentially need if we decided to move in that direction?

Chapter 12

THE MAGIC TRICK

In this, the last chapter, I want to explain the erotic magic trick our bodies are capable of that liberates us to explore the wildest, most joyful aspects of living. I call it a "magic trick" because that's what it felt like when I stumbled into it in my early twenties. In the decades since, I've learned about the physiological and neurobiological underpinnings of it. All that science means I could write about it like I'm writing about a "biohack," a way of manipulating the mechanisms of your embodied mind to make it do something really cool. The science behind this, mostly grounded in interpersonal neuroscience, is amazing, but it is not what I'm going to talk about in this chapter, because thinking about it as a way to hack your body will not get you there. Instead, I'll suggest you think of it as a *way of knowing* through erotic wisdom.

But let's start with a definition. What do I mean by "erotic"?

It's Been Your Aliveness, All Along

Audre Lorde wrote, "I speak of the erotic as the deepest life force, a force which moves us toward living in a fundamental way."

Ask anyone who had to pee for hours before they finally got relief. Ask anyone who went days without food and then took their first bite. Ask any runner who gets home from a long, hot run and chugs water straight from the tap, then palms more water onto their face and throat and arms. The physical experience of meeting our bodies' needs is also an emotional experience and a sensuous experience. It is *erotic*.

Throughout this book I've been saying "erotic energy" and "erotic connection" for a reason. I don't just mean sexual connection. I mean life itself.

Lorde wrote in her essay "Uses of the Erotic":

The erotic is a measure between the beginnings of our sense of self and the chaos of our strongest feelings. It is an internal sense of satisfaction to which, once we have experienced it, we know we can aspire. For having experienced the fullness of this depth of feeling and recognizing its power, in honor and self-respect we can require no less of ourselves. . . . Once we know the extent to which we are capable of feeling that sense of satisfaction and completion, we can then observe which of our various life endeavors bring us closest to that fullness.

You live in a body. That body needs things from the world in order for it to stay balanced enough to support life. It needs to take in air from the world, it needs to take in water. We need the microscopic organisms that call us home; they make it possible for us to digest the food that itself was once alive and dependent on the Earth, just as we are. And human bodies of all ages and abilities need at least some tender connection.

One of the ways we get that connection is through sex. And

that's erotic. But we can also get that connection need met through hugs and massage, through eye contact and smiles, through playing together, working together, singing, laughing, praying, or dancing together. All of that is erotic, too, if we allow ourselves to notice how our bodies resonate with life force when we accept from the world these resources we need in order to stay alive.

"Am I alive? I'm alive. This is what it feels like to be alive." That is the doorway to the erotic. It replaces all the imperatives that would have us look away from our own internal experience; it guides us back to who we truly are.

A lot of people whose bodies and sexualities defy the handbooks they were given at birth already have practice at ignoring the rules and choosing for themselves. LGBTQIA2+ folks, BIPOC folks, lots of disabled or neurodivergent folks, fat folks, and aging folks may already know that you can choose what you like, outside the limited offerings of the sex imperatives. In this book, I wanted to offer tools all of us can use to return to our erotic selves, no matter how the world has tried to control, erase, or diminish us, our aliveness.

Not everything about being alive in a body feels magical or even pleasurable. But we can increase our brain's access to the pleasurable parts of being alive by practicing a skill called "savoring."

Start with Savoring

A large and growing focus in positive psychology is on the phenomenon of savoring, which, in its technical sense, refers to people's "capacity to attend to, appreciate, and enhance the positive feelings in their lives."[1] As researchers measure it, we take mental snapshots of positive moments, using a particular set of strategies, to enhance our awareness and memory of positive moments. The strategies, delineated in the Savoring Checklist, include:[2]

- *Sharing with Others.* In the moment, we talk to someone with whom we're sharing the experience, or tell others how much we value the moment. This translates well to an erotic experience shared with a partner. Saying out loud how much we are enjoying an experience while we're having it, or how much we enjoyed it or how meaningful it was, right after, amplifies the pleasure and solidifies it in our memory.

- *Temporal Awareness.* Time is our most valuable resource because it is the only thing we have that, once it's gone, we can never have again. Our body's energy can be renewed, money comes and goes, but time is limited and fleeting. Temporal awareness is reminding ourselves how transient time is and therefore noticing this moment, cherishing it before it passes. This is an easy savoring behavior to integrate into an erotic experience. "Time is short, and I choose to do *this* with my time."

- *Behavioral Expression.* This refers to the way we enact our positive emotions. We laugh out loud, jump up and down, clap our hands and whoop. We allow our bodies to be so full of the pleasure of the moment that we can't help flapping our hands in excitement. If we have pleasure shame, as so many of us do, this is a great strategy for cracking open the shell of shame and letting our pleasure fly free. Practicing behavioral expression of positive emotions outside of a sexual context will make it more natural within a sexual context.

- *Sensory-Perceptual Sharpening.* This might be the strategy people are most likely to think of when they think of "mindfulness." We slow down and pay attention to a specific sensation or group of sensations, to the exclusion of everything else. We allow our attention to focus on the sensations around our genitals. Or just notice the sensation of your partner's mouth on yours, shutting out the whole world.

There's an anti-savoring skill, too, with which we are all too familiar: *Killjoy Thinking*. These are the thoughts we have in the midst of enjoyment, to remind ourselves of all the other things we should be doing ("Sure, we got ourselves into the bed and naked, but there's still a sink full of dishes!"), or to critique the ways this positive event could or should have been better ("The sex was enjoyable, but my partner didn't have an orgasm—they didn't *want* an orgasm, but still . . ."), or to dwell on what a struggle it was to get to this positive moment ("Finally, we're here, but ugh, what a hassle it was, the negotiation and checking in and all those *feelings* . . .").

Some people consider savoring pleasure to be an "indulgence." Rather than really enjoying the pleasure they experience, they furtively sneak the pleasure in, quick and stolen, rather than expansive and fully owned. Savoring versus sneaking is the difference between a leisurely, candlelit masturbation session where you touch every part of your body and allow pleasure to ebb and flow like an incoming tide, versus a two-minute wank in the shower before work. Neither is a bad way to experience pleasure, as long as you are free of guilt or shame. But savoring brings with it an extra set of benefits:

First, the practice of attending to, appreciating, and enhancing positive feelings can increase the amount of pleasure that we *remember.* If pleasure is the shy animal I described back in chapter 2, then savoring is a way of taking a mental snapshot or a tiny looping video of the inner animal of our pleasure, rolling around in the grass. Locking pleasure in to our memories through savoring is a skill worth learning, not least because we make our decisions today not so much based on rational pros and cons of a given choice, but based on our memories of the past. To help us choose pleasure in the future, it helps if we remember the pleasure of the past. When we habitually capture the pleasure of the present moment, then the next time we have an opportunity to choose between the easy but bland pleasure of a familiar TV show versus the more effortful but more delicious and potentially more meaningful pleasure of an erotic encounter with our partner, our brains remember how worth it the extra effort is.

But wait, there's more! As time management expert Laura Vanderkam describes in *Off the Clock*, when we savor pleasure and thus highlight it in our memory, we can remember our lives as *more worth living*. We look back on our day, our year, even our entire lifetime, and we see less of the struggle and more of the countless moments of pleasure, from the tiny pleasures of the meal you savored last night or the shower you prolonged to enjoy the water on your skin, to the vast, overwhelming pleasures of meeting your child for the first time, falling in love, or, after you give a TED Talk, seeing three thousand people rise to their feet, hearing the sound of their applause, feeling in your body that you did something right. All of these glitter across our memory, brighter and more numerous, when we take time to savor them.

Start with savoring. It is a powerful antidote to pleasure shame, but, even more, it leads to a life well lived.

Erotic Wisdom

In the previous chapter, I advised women in heterosexual-type relationships to acknowledge the part of them that is wise, the part that does not either fall into the old, well-worn habits of a Giver or react with anger against a Winner. Both the habits and the anger are real and they are parts of all of us, and we will inevitably spend a lot of time with those parts as we gradually find our way out of scripted instruction-manual sex imperatives and gender stuff, and into a sexuality that is authentically our own, vulnerable, curious, autonomous, and welcome. We will bounce from noticing that we're following the handbook to reacting against the handbook to looking to ourselves and our partners for what's true. That third process, looking to ourselves and our partners for what's true, is erotic wisdom.

So I want you to get to know this part of you that is wise. You meet this part not through any rational, scientific process, but by accessing your erotic way of knowing—that is, through your body and imagination.

So as you're sitting comfortably, with your hands relaxed and, if it feels right, with your eyes closed, I'd like to you to take a deep, slow breath in . . .

And I'd like you to release that breath even more slowly.

And again, take a deep, slow breath in . . . And a slow, slow breath out.

As you're breathing you can be aware of any tension in your abdominal muscles and in your thoracic diaphragm, right under your lungs, just let that soften. Let your belly be spacious.

Deep, deep, deep in your core, your pelvic diaphragm that runs from your tailbone down in a sling of muscle through your genitals to your pubic bone. Just let it sink right down. And any unnecessary tension you find in any of those muscles, you can just let go, as you continue to breathe deeply and slowly.

As you open up all this space inside you, you begin to notice a pleasant, quiet light glowing deep in your core. And that warm, quiet glow begins to grow in that peaceful space you've created inside yourself. The more the light spreads, the more you begin to feel your body resonating with an intense, quiet joy that expands inside you as you continue breathing, deeply and slowly. And that joyful light spreads through your whole belly and all through your heart, and fills up your whole torso, and continues to grow as you breathe deeply and slowly. This quiet light filling your arms and legs, enveloping your spine, all the way up to your skull and filling your whole head with this blissful, peaceful, joyful light.

Sitting here, still breathing deeply and slowly, feeling so filled with quiet and peace, you know that this is a feeling and a place inside yourself that you can return to at any time. A safe and tranquil place that you carry inside you always.

And as you're continuing to breathe deeply and slowly, I'd like you to allow the inner screen of your mind, that's usually so noisy and crowded, to grow comparatively quiet and blank and calm. You'll notice thoughts that want to move onto your inner screen and get your attention. Just notice them, know that you can return to that thought at another time, and let them stroll on by. Let your inner screen grow a little quieter and a little calmer. If your mind is like mine, it may never be entirely silent or still, and that's okay, too. We're just slowing things down some, turning down the volume, to create some space, the way you created space in your belly.

On this quiet, calm screen, as you're breathing deeply and slowly, I'd like you to allow to emerge: your inner guide.

It might show up as someone you know personally.

It might be someone you don't know.

It might be a fictional character or someone from history.

Or it might be an animal.

Whomever you most need to hear from is who will emerge.

Right now, this guide is a part of your own mind, your own internal sage, an expert on you and your heart and your sexuality, who will answer any question you ask, as long as you continue breathing, slowly and deeply.

While you're in this safe space with your guide, you can ask any question you like.

You might ask:

What do I need?

Where am I going?

Who am I, really?

When do I love myself most?

When is it easiest for me to be compassionate?

For the next five minutes, still breathing deeply and slowly, you can chat with your guide and find out what you need to know.

After five minutes, or whenever you're ready, join me again.

You're still sitting comfortably and breathing deeply and slowly, and you know that you can come back and talk with your guide whenever you want to, because you carry them inside you always, in this safe, quiet place. I'd like you to allow yourself a gathering awareness of your body in the room, and of your hands, and your heart. Know that everything that happens from now until you go to bed tonight will be touched by the peace and joy you bring with you into the room as you allow yourself a gathering awareness of your shoulders and your head and face, and are aware now of your belly and still feeling that quiet, steady joy, aware of your legs and of your feet and now of your eyelids, which, if they're closed, whenever you're ready, you can open.

I've been leading an inner guide meditation like this for about three decades. Sometimes people just fall asleep, and that's fine, too, because sleep is important. But if they stay awake, almost everyone finds themselves in conversation with someone who knows their strengths and their struggles and always keeps their best interests at heart. A kind and patient someone, who somehow lives inside them and yet knows more than they themselves do. This inner wisdom isn't mind and it isn't body; it is the erotic itself. It is aliveness.

The Magic Trick: What It Is

So what is the magic trick, what does it feel like, and how does it work?

The magic trick surfaces the erotic wisdom inside you and creates a context that allows your erotic wisdom to merge with others. Simple enough, right? Heh.

In his book on Internal Family Systems, *No Bad Parts,* Richard Schwartz writes about a "field of SELF," as a different way of experiencing Self, our sense of individual existence in connection with others. He writes:

> *Quantum physics tells us that a photon is both a particle and a wave. I believe the same is true for the Self. Most of the time we experience Self in its particle state—we feel some degree of connectedness to others and SELF while also sensing that we are separate entities with boundaries and individual agency. Through meditation or psychedelics, however, we can lose those boundaries and enter the wave state—we become part of the much larger field of Self (SELF) in a way that feels numinous. . . .*
>
> *We already know about magnetic or gravitational fields, but as [theoretical physicist Sean] Carroll points out, "The universe is full of fields, and what we think of as particles are just excitations of those fields, like waves in an ocean."*

. . . I believe there is a field of Self. We can enter that field through meditation, for example, and become part of that field and lose our particle-ness.

I believe the "magic trick," as I call it, is actually access to the field of SELF.

In fact, as I read about that field, a cross between physics and spirituality, I thought of the Rumi poem:

Out beyond ideas of wrongdoing and rightdoing, there is a field. I'll meet you there.

What if we could find ourselves in an uncultivated, uncultivatable field, where our sense of individual existence melts away and all the rules we have ever followed simply do not apply? There is no "you" separate from your beloved, there is only YOU, together, playing in a field of US, all of us, the unity that is the human spirit.

Do I think there's an actual, literal field of SELF, like a magnetic field or gravitational field?

¯_(ツ)_/¯

But I know there's a place I can go where I experience exactly what Richard Schwartz describes as his own and his patients' experiences.

You might be familiar with the quote "Any sufficiently advanced technology is indistinguishable from magic." What I'm describing is a technology of human aliveness itself.

If you are alive in a body, no matter what else is true about that body, it's true that you have access to the magic. The magic is a field, in every sense.

What does it feel like?

It feels like your individual self disappears or diminishes or dissolves or melts into the other people. It feels like your individual self expands to encompass the larger You. You feel bigger. You feel as if you, as you, barely exist. You feel still and at peace. You feel restless with ever-expanding energy. I've talked to several hundred people who've experienced it, and here are just a few of their descriptions:

It feels like god or Love takes me completely. . . . It's like I become one of those multifaceted suncatcher crystals for a moment and the light moves through me. I feel, for a moment, like I am connected to everything on Earth. Like the ocean and the leaves in the trees and the stretch and breath of animals and movement of wind and rain and microbes are all part of me. This is what I mean by I feel god, I feel that I am held by and in and with all life. It is both powerful and humbling and often brings tears of joy.

It feels like I'm floating in the universe. I see stars, sounds fade a bit, my skin is SUPER sensitive (in a good way!), and I can't stop giggling.

It feels like I am connected to some sacred energy source in the universe, and at the same time, I am deeply connected with and in harmony with my spouse.

Sometimes you have an orgasm, too. The actual physiology of the orgasm may all but vanish in the midst of the hugeness of the magic trick.

Seem like something you might want to try? Let's talk about how.

The Magic Trick: How To

How do you do it? Here's my formula, to achieve the magic trick: Move your body in time with others, for a shared purpose, by choice.

1. *Move your body.* As a technology of human aliveness, the magic trick is about embodiment, exploring your body as a location of erotic ecstasy. Moving it is a powerful way to facilitate and sustain contact with your erotic wisdom.

2. *In time.* Did you know that when toddlers bounce in rhythm with an adult, it increases their cooperative be-

havior with that adult? Our bodies automatically shift their biological rhythms, to move in time with the bodies of the people around us. That scene in *Dead Poets Society,* where the boys shift from strolling around at their own pace to marching in step together? That's a real phenomenon called "entrainment." You may have experienced it yourself in a dance class, a choir, or a community hike. Sure it can be used as a weapon, but it can also be used as a bridge that leads to the field of SELF.

3. *With others.* Erotic connection in a long-term relationship is different from other erotic experiences, because it is the co-creation of a shared space. You bring your bodies into a shared space that you cultivate together.

4. *For a shared purpose.* The very first question we asked at the start of this book was "Is sex important?" Each of us has to answer that question for ourselves, for any given relationship and in any given season of our lives. The answer changes. And when sex is important, we can further ask: Why *this* sex? What is it for? Where is it taking you?— you alone or you together with a partner.

5. *By choice.* The magic trick is always voluntary. The magic trick doesn't happen through force or a sense of either obligation or entitlement.

Of these five components, the only one that's absolutely mandatory is . . . did you guess? Yes. It's "by choice." If you have that one, you can probably do the magic trick with any combination of three others. You don't have to move your body, necessarily. You don't have to have a shared purpose necessarily. You don't have to be with others, necessarily. You don't have to create a rhythm intentionally.

The magic trick happens in a context of expanding freedom. It is curious exploration. It is play. It is everything in all the chapters that led to this one; it is everything in all the moments of your life that led to this one.

I hope you notice that the magic trick does not by any means have to be a sexual experience. My sister experiences it singing in a group. I've experienced it swing dancing with a partner. During one particularly excellent lindy hop, somebody walked by me and my partner and muttered, "Get a room." What he and I were doing was *erotic,* and this passerby misinterpreted it as sexual. I've also experienced it cycling along a rural hillside, alone. I've experienced it masturbating alone, as well as during sex with a partner. I've gotten really close, too, in moments, while sitting at my computer writing this book.

You may experience it praying with others in a worship service, marching in a protest, laughing with friends, playing a team sport, or as you work on an art project. The magic trick accesses the erotic, your very aliveness, not merely your sexuality. Practicing it outside of sex might even make it more accessible during sex!

Practice the Magic, Solo

For some people, this is a spiritual practice. For some, it is a therapeutic practice. For some, it's literally an accident, something they stumble on without realizing what they've found. That's what it was for me, the first time; now it's a love practice, a ritual I can share with my long-term partner, to lead us up a mountain to a place where we might find something unlike anything else on Earth.

Your task, with this practice, is to let your body and your awareness of your body *take up space*. In an erotic context, especially in a sexual context, "taking up space" asks you to do something that might feel counterintuitive: soften. Be at ease, in the midst of tension.

The cycle of sexual arousal involves an increase in physical tension in your body, generated in response to sex-related stimulation. Orgasm itself is the spontaneous, involuntary release of that tension, so a lot of advice for having an orgasm or even creating intense sexual pleasure says you should *increase* tension.

But the magic trick calls for ease. Allow yourself to be in your body, to notice where tension is accumulating and then soften the edges of that tension, so that it spreads out. The tension doesn't disappear; it's just the same amount of tension, spread over a larger area in your body. And when you're with a partner, that tension expands not just within your body but also into the space between you and your partner.

So, rather than letting the tension accumulate just in your genitals, you inhale with a soft belly, notice the tension, and exhale, allowing that tension to dissipate out from your genitals across your whole pelvis. Then you accumulate more tension, with more stimulation. And again, you inhale with a soft belly as you notice all that tension building up in your genitals and across your whole pelvis, and then exhale and allow that tension to dissipate across your thighs and belly.

Again and again, you let the tension gently fill you up. It won't feel like the typical tension that precedes a typical orgasm, where your muscles may be locked up and rigid, your breath held tight in your lungs. Instead, it will feel more like waves that move through you with your breath. This is the natural rhythm of your body.

If you want to dive deep into experiencing what it is to live in your body, you could start with Ev'Yan Whitney's beautiful book of guided journaling, *Sensual Self: Prompts and Practices for Getting in Touch with Your Body*. It offers dozens of embodiment practices and reflection. Nearly all of them will work for asexual folks, because the focus is on sensuality, literally the sensations of the body, not on sexuality, which appears in moments and nudges but not as a central theme. One of my favorite prompts begins with this guidance:

> *Choose a part of your body—the top of your head, your pinky toe, your left elbow, the roof of your mouth—and bring con-*

scious awareness to it. See if you can feel into that specific part of your body, isolating it from all others. Bring focus and awareness to the aliveness of this part of your body.

You can also start by focusing on the pleasure of one partner at a time. Caress and kiss and stimulate your partner, allow pleasure to grow in their body, and then create space between you, allow their pleasure to dissipate. If they're experiencing genital arousal, let that arousal ease. Let a penis lose its erection. Let a vulva diminish its swelling. Then touch your partner again. It can help to begin your touch at the periphery of their body—fingertips and toes and scalp—and gradually, in wave after wave of stimulation, shift your attention and touch body parts closer and closer to their core. I'm talking about extravagant amounts of time spent on allowing pleasure and arousal to grow and dissipate, grow and dissipate. Half an hour, an hour, more.

And then next time you and your partner connect erotically, switch roles.

Eventually, the person receiving stimulation may get to a place that feels close to orgasm or the edge of . . . something. It will become increasingly counterintuitive to stop stimulation, to allow tension to dissipate. Your body will want something, to go somewhere.

When you get to that feeling, slow down even more. You're nearing the peak, and if you can be still inside yourself, breathing and easeful in the midst of the delicious chaos of intense, long-lasting arousal and pleasure, you might blip into the field.

If you don't . . . well, the worst thing that could happen is you experience extended erotic pleasure. Oh no, too bad. 😊

Ama and Di

I'd like to conclude our story of Ama and Di with a time Di used the magic trick.

"How 'bout I go down on you for a while this afternoon?" Di asked over breakfast, the morning after their first night in a long time when they got to be alone in the house to-

gether. The night had been sex-free, Ama too exhausted to focus on the delicious meal Di had cooked, much less on erotic touch. They had made a lot of headway on a thousand-piece jigsaw puzzle, though, and made up a lot of word games.

At Di's suggestion of oral sex, Ama smiled and shrugged. "Sounds good. Low pressure."

What she didn't know was that Di's "for a while" meant "about an hour and a half." After a lazy shower together, they got into bed and Di began not with Ama's genitals but with her periphery—her fingertips and the palms of her hands, her toes and the soles of her feet. The insides of her elbows and the backs of her knees. Her armpits, the curve where her ear meets her jaw, the undercurve of her breasts, the undercurve of her belly. Ama was humming and sighing with pleasure by the time Di got anywhere near her clitoris.

After a very short time attending to Ama's clit, Di paused and lay beside her and they whispered to each other about what they liked most about each other and their relationship. Then Di said, "Ready for a little more?"

Ama nodded, and Di began again, not quite at the beginning, but spending time with Ama's breasts, bum, and belly before she got back to the genitals. She stayed a while, and Ama, freed from any expectation or performance demand, allowed her arousal to grow slowly. Eventually, her abdominal muscles began to tremble with tension . . . and Di paused again, lying beside her again and chatting with her about this and that, little things, pleasant things. What they might have for dinner. How well the parlor palm was growing in its new spot by the northeast-facing window. She touched Ama all the while, stroking her hand over Ama's torso and arms and thighs. Ama's arousal faded to a light warmth inside her.

Then Di began again, and Ama's arousal grew again, and Di paused again. Once more, Ama's arousal faded as

Di kissed her neck and whispered the funny sweet nothings they had shared for so many years.

Ama breathed a laugh and said, "I'm sorry, I feel like all my arousal is just draining away and you have to start over."

"Well yeah," Di said matter-of-factly. "I'm doing that on purpose."

"Oh," Ama said, and she put her hands over her face. "That's really hot."

"I thought so!" Di answered with a laugh, and she returned her mouth to Ama's clitoris.

The benefit of taking it slow is that arousal has time to grow in every part of your body, not just in the parts we usually associate with sexual arousal. Ama spends a lot of her life in CARE and FEAR, and she rarely has an opportunity to allow her whole brain to disengage from the concerns of her life and family and settle comfortably into LUST.

Each time Di stopped, Ama's brain had the opportunity to slip out of LUST and maybe into an adverse space, but Di stayed close to her—close with her body, close with her voice, close with her affection—so Ama never drifted too far, always going no further than CARE and PLAY. Di's intention was to put no clock on it, to allow pleasure to grow as it wanted. Once Ama knew what Di was doing and knew Di was succeeding even more than she realized, Ama got a serious case of the giggles. She wanted to explain what made her laugh, but every time she tried to speak, she burst into another fit of mirth. The laughter grew along with her arousal, and Di laughed, too, even as she kept her mouth on her partner, and Di's laughter touched Ama and made her laugh more, and turned her on more, and her body rode the tide of pleasure and joy to the shores of something she had always suspected might exist but had never experienced. A kind of floating, shimmering bliss. Quiet, like a breeze in trees, only it was her own breath and Di's.

It's the kind of thing they say in romance novels, right?

"Riding the tide of pleasure to the shores of blah blah blah . . ." It's silly. I hear it, too. But this is a true story.

I'm telling you, friends, it exists. It might not be someplace you can go to in your current season of life; maybe you might never have a chance to get there. But just knowing it's there, knowing you might . . . isn't that what hope feels like? And even if you and your partner spend the time you have together just daydreaming about it, that's all it takes to bring it a little closer.

Take your time. Stay connected and present. And practice, practice, practice. Good things come.

The Magic Trick: Why, Though?

If you're a reader like me, maybe you skipped the other chapters and went right to this one. Like, *"Let's just get to the ecstasy part,"* right?

Alas, alas.

You have to climb Pleasure Mountain.

Sex researcher Shemeka Thorpe, in her research on Black women's pleasure, used the metaphor of "Pleasure Mountain," with a collection of tools and landmarks that her research participants used to climb it.[3]

Similarly, the cover of Peggy Kleinplatz and Dana Ménard's book, *Magnificent Sex,* features a big mountain with the sun behind it, because the metaphor they found themselves working with was a mountain. In their research on "Optimal Sexual Experiences" (OSEs) and the "magnificent lovers" who experience them, the team found that the magnificent lovers climbed many different paths to reach the top of that mountain.

"From the peak of the mountain," they write, "the view is always superb; however the pathways to the mountaintop are hardly uniform—they are unique."[4]

It's probably not a coincidence that the two most compelling recent research projects on sexual pleasure both center the experiences of people whose sexuality is often marginalized—older people, kinky people, and nonmonogamous people in the case of the OSE research, and Black women in the South, in the case of Shemeka Thorpe and her team. And in both the OSE research and the Black women's sexuality's research, the metaphor of the mountain is prominent.

The "trick" of the magic trick isn't that you can magically transport yourself or your partner to a peak of ecstasy, nor can your partner magically transport you. You have to climb. You probably have to climb the mountain over and over again, exploring different paths, attempting different climbing styles. Maybe you're walking up a switchback trail, maybe you're scrambling with your hands and feet, maybe you're tied in on a rope looped through an anchor in the rock, left behind for you by some previous climber, and your partner is belaying you.

Sound like a lot of effort? You're not wrong!

Let me repeat: You never have to. This is a bonus extra, for people interested in experiencing a shared erotic wisdom, a sense of aliveness that transports them out of their individual existence into a space of, well, magic.

So *why* climb the mountain? What exactly do people find up there?

Just as I've asked hundreds of people to tell me what it is they want when they want sex, I've asked hundreds more to tell me what benefit ecstasy has in their lives. And just as people overwhelmingly say they want connection, people overwhelmingly say that the magic trick brings them connection: Connection with a partner. Connection with their own bodies. And connection to something larger than themselves, the thing I call the field and they called "the universe," "the ultimate source," "the answer," "creation," and, well, "magic."

Connection with a Partner:

Feeling 100 percent connected to and loved by my partner, which enables me to feel more loving and compassionate in my everyday life.

It improved our already really intense connection. It brought in the ability to have discussions about that and a lot of other things in a new, extra vulnerable way. Everything feels fully surrendered, and the trust is unlike anything ever experienced or seen elsewhere before.

Connection with My Body:

It releases me from the near-constant experience of fear I have in my body, if only for a little bit. It lets me glimpse what physical relaxation really is. It also gives me experiences of sexuality and my own body that really feel safe. After sexual trauma and a long period totally disconnected from my body, these heightened sexual experiences have helped me start to reconnect with sexuality as both a thing that is safe and a thing that is part of me.

It has a specific medicinal quality for me: I live with daily pain from a spine injury/rebuild, and an immune disease that requires painful weekly treatment, so my baseline experience in my own flesh can be a bit beleaguered in the day-to-day: I actually really need a thriving athletic life and a thriving sexual life to "balance" the experiences of pain and difficulty in my body with experiences of endorphins, oxytocin, etc.—but also experiences of success, joy, and congruence between who I am and how my body will express that, so sexual ecstasy is something I prioritize, prize, nurture. [This idea of pain management/physical healing is common in narratives of disabled people in The Bump'n Book of Love, Lust & Disability.*]*[5]

Connection with the Field:

I feel like I have a superpower. On really bad days, knowing that I have this ability to feel really good can get me through hard things, like knowing you have a hefty savings account, or a secret stash of amazing chocolate cake that no one else knows about that you can tap into when you want it. It makes life sweeter and connects me to hope in the face of fatigue and all of the suffering in the world. It brings me gratitude and joy and amazement that my body and being can do this after all of the trauma I have experienced.

My spiritual awakening was closely tied to sexual ecstasy. It makes me feel more deeply connected not just to my partner, but to all of creation. I consider sexual ecstasy to be divine, and it is an important (though rare) spiritual practice in my life.

This is something much bigger than sex, bigger even than pleasure. I think finding your way to the magic field changes people, enhances their connection to their own inner wisdom, grants them more consistent access to kindness and compassion. If you have the time, energy, and emotional wherewithal to try it, I believe you will find that it makes you a better person, and makes your relationship a force for good in the world.

It will look unique on your body and on your partner's body and on everyone's bodies, the way yoga looks different on everyone's bodies. Not everyone can put their legs behind their heads to practice advanced yoga postures—some people's anatomy just isn't built for it. But putting your legs behind your head is not the yoga; stretching your body in the direction of the posture, that's the yoga. Stretch your sexuality in the direction of the magic. If you make your way all the way to the magical field, super! Neat! But even if you "only" move ever closer to it . . . I mean, wow.

Wow.

Astonishing changes can happen in your life, just because you reached for the magic.

But again: Bonus extra! Never mandatory! There are no "imperatives" in this book, apart from consent. There are only tools and maps and seeds to plant.

Chapter 12 tl;dr:

- Practice savoring pleasure in all domains of life by sharing it with others, focusing your sensory awareness on it, expressing it with your body, and other strategies.

- Through something similar to guided meditation, connect with the part of yourself that is wise, the part that knows the answers to any questions you have. This is a way of knowing the world that allows you to feel most alive.

- The "magic trick" for accessing ecstasy involves moving your body in time with other people, for a shared purpose, with mutual consent. You can practice it with a partner or solo—you might find it easier solo at first.

- Why practice ecstasy? Because it's not just about sex; it's about your aliveness. It can deepen your connection with a partner, but it can also lead you to something larger, a sense of connection with what it means to be alive in a human body.

Some Good Questions:

- What's it like to connect with my erotic wisdom?

- What time, attention, or energy might be worth investing in the magic trick? What might change in my

life, that could change the time, attention, or energy
I can invest?

- What obstacles stand between me and reaching for
the magic?

- What happens in my body when I'm exploring the
erotic unknown?

CONCLUSION

In any relationship that lasts long enough, it is not just normal, it is *inevitable* that there will be a time when partners have different levels of interest in sex, different sexual experiences they're interested in having, and different abilities to be sexual. Normal. Not a problem. I've been through it myself, and I've used the tools in this book to find my way back to my certain special someone. For us, the "What If?" Daydream to rebuild emotional accessibility and a deeper grappling with my training as a Giver were the most essential parts of the process, along with the foundational tools of confidence and joy, admiration and trust, calm, warm curiosity, and the emotional floorplan. When this book is published and I start traveling again, we'll probably have another dry spell, but now I know for sure that we will always be able to find our way back to each other. You can have that, too.

The most efficient way to turn that normal, inevitable season into a problem is to worry about it. The sex imperatives and the gender mirage want you to worry, want you to believe that something bad could happen if you jettison their rules and wholeheartedly embrace who you truly are, as you are right now. That's why sometimes joy—loving what's true—can feel scary, like jumping off a cliff in the dark, with no idea what will happen next.

But isn't that just like life? We step into each new day with no guarantee of what will come next, only a commitment to make of the day and our lives something worth remembering. Our only certainty is that one day, we won't get any more days.

Over the years that I was writing this book, a friend in her sixties had a stroke, my twin had a serious medical diagnosis, multiple in-laws had serious medical diagnoses, and *I* had a serious medical diagnosis. And just as I was finishing the book, my friend Anna died. She was in her forties, around my age, and she and her wife had been married just ten years. She was a librarian and a fiber artist and an activist, and I loved her. It's unfair and enraging and a cavernous, harrowing loss. Also: Fuck cancer.

But Anna always said, "Queer joy matters. Stay safe, stay fierce, practice hope." And so, in the face of the life-altering, life-threatening, and life-ending events that happen every day, we practice hope at my house, and we practice pleasure. Life is too short and too uncertain to have sex you don't like—or, at the very least, aren't really curious to try.

Couples who sustain a strong sexual connection over the long term are different from each other in myriad ways, but in one way they are all the same: They collaborate to create a context that makes pleasure easier to access, not least by turning toward each other's whole, authentic selves with confidence, joy, and calm, warm curiosity.

Be who you truly are, safe in a connection where all of you is welcome. Love who you love. Love *how* you love.

Will other people have opinions? Sure.

Keep weeding the garden.

Come Together tl;dr:

1. Pleasure is the measure of sexual well-being—not how much you want it, how often you do it, with whom, where, what time of day, or even whether you have orgasms. It's whether or not you like the sex you are having. Life is too short to have sex you don't like.

2. Pleasure is sensation in context—a sensation you experience in a stressful context may feel uncomfortable, while the same sensation in a great, sexy context may feel pleasurable. Context is both your external circumstances and your internal state. Your external circumstances include everything from your relationship to your culture, including the sex imperatives and the gender mirage. Your internal state includes everything in your emotional floorplan, including the bonus spaces of your THINKING MIND and OBSERVATIONAL DISTANCE, plus the state of your physical body.

3. Couples who sustain a strong sexual connection over the long term co-create a context that makes pleasure easier to access. They treat their shared context as a "third thing," a joint project or hobby toward which they both feel enthusiasm and investment. Treating it as a shared project on which you and your partner collaborate helps you avoid falling into blame traps, where a sexual difficulty is one person's fault. Instead, a difficulty is always a result of a problem with the context, which you can adjust together.

4. Your emotional floorplan includes pleasure-favorable spaces—LUST, SEEKING, PLAY, and CARE—and pleasure-adverse spaces—FEAR, RAGE, and PANIC/GRIEF. Map out your emotional floorplans to see why sometimes it's easy

to get to a sexy state of mind and sometimes it's impossible. It will also help you to understand and articulate ways to make it easier for each other to get to the spaces adjacent to LUST.

5. Certain sex-positive mindsets allow you to cultivate a shared garden. First, confidence—knowing what's true—and joy—loving what's true—are the keys to creating the sex life that's a great fit for you and your relationship. Second, reconceive changes and differences in sexuality not as a linear progression from broken → normal → perfect but as an ongoing cycle of woundedness to healing, and you're already perfect, wherever you are within that cycle. These tools can free you to turn toward your sexuality and your erotic connection with kindness and compassion.

6. The foundational tools of a great relationship are trust—which is made of emotional accessibility, emotional responsiveness, and emotional engagement—and admiration. Recognizing admirable traits can help you choose a partner worth staying with, and remembering admirable traits in a long-term partner can help motivate you to work through whatever difficulty you may face.

7. Together with the science of behavior change, calm, warm curiosity is the most important tool for solving problems. Curiosity will allow you to address the realities of living in bodies that change with time and even solve the tricky problems that arise in long-term connections, such as "How do I get my partner on board with change?" and "How do we move past old hurts?"

8. The "sex imperatives" want you to feel an urgent impulse to change your individual sexuality and your sexual connection, to make it more like what it "should" be.

Don't fall for it. No sexual difficulty is worth damaging a great relationship.

9. Perhaps the most ubiquitous and the most insidious barrier between us and our full erotic potential is the "gender mirage"—the idea that because you were born with a particular set of body parts, there are highly specific rules you must obey about how to live in that body and be a sexual person. Heterosexual-type relationships might struggle the most with the gender mirage, since the relationship does not inherently contradict the rules of the mirage.

10. When we collaborate to co-create a context that makes pleasure easy, not just by addressing our external circumstances (including the sex imperatives and the gender mirage), but by learning to navigate our own and our partners' emotional floorplans, we gain access to what I call "the magic trick," a state of ecstasy that connects us to the larger meaning of living a human life.

APPENDIX 1

Ten "But, Emily!" Questions

1. But, Emily, I just want my partner to have more sex with me. How do I get my partner to have more sex with me?
Reread chapter 1 and consider the more specific question, "What is it that I want when I want more sex with my partner?" (Hint: It's not orgasm, you can probably do that on your own.) You might also discuss with your partner what it is they *don't* want when they don't want more sex with you.

Do you believe you need the sex? Please visit The "It's a Boy!" Handbook in chapter 10 (not because you're a boy, necessarily, but because that's where I mention that sex is not a biological need whose absence can cause you harm). For more details see chapter 7 of *Come as You Are.*

This is also an excellent moment to revisit chapter 6, regarding admiration. Recalling what you find admirable about your partner can help recalibrate your attention away from your frustration and back toward the human you chose and who chose you.

Also, just a quick reminder that sex is not something we "get" other people to do, it's an experience we co-create by choice. Is what you want when you want more sex with your partner, for your partner to be there reluctantly?

2. But, Emily, I just want my partner to stop hassling me for sex. How do I get them to stop hassling me?

I highly recommend saying something like "Please stop hassling me for sex." You might add, "Hassling hits my brakes and makes it even more difficult for me to want or like sex." You might even say, "Let's have a conversation about what it is you want when you want sex, and what it is I don't want when I don't want sex." It's a rich starting place for a great deal of conversation and mutual learning, if you can avoid treating sex like a power struggle (see chapter 11) and instead like a mutual hobby and shared pleasure.

You can also point them to question 1 in this appendix.

3. But where am I supposed to get the time/energy/motivation required to create a context that grants my brain access to pleasure?

It's a strange new phenomenon, people asking me, "How am I supposed to want/like/have sex under these adverse circumstances?" Just since the pandemic, really, people have asked me, not rhetorically, "How am I supposed to do this?" It feels to me like something shifted in the cultural discourse around sexuality, where people—maybe especially women—feel obliged to be sexual, regardless of the context.

And of course the answer is: You're not. You're not supposed to. If your life circumstances—your stress level, your responsibilities, your relationship, your health, both physical and mental—are just not compatible with creating a context that makes pleasure easier to access, that's just what's true for you in this season of your life. I wish it weren't true for you, for your sake. I think no one who loves you would want you to stay in that state longer than absolutely necessary. But we don't always get to decide what's happening in our lives and relationships.

I can say, though, that if you and a partner collaborate to change those circumstances, or if a partner really steps up to make those circumstances less onerous, you might discover that energy is freed up for pleasure.

4. But what if talking about sex is a turn-off? I know I'm supposed to believe consent is sexy or whatever, but I (or my partner) feel like being *asked* for something makes it more difficult to say yes, or if I have to ask, it feels like my partner isn't paying enough attention.
This question is so hard to answer, not because it's complicated but because nobody ever feels satisfied by the truth.

Ask yourself (and/or your partner): What is it about talking about sex that hits the brakes?

Do you feel that you shouldn't have to? Then of course it hits the brakes! If you believe talking means there's something wrong, that judgment, like most judgment, is going to hit the brakes.

Do you believe your partner should already know what you want, or that you should be able to tell what a partner wants, without having to communicate about it? Then, once again, of course it hits the brakes.

Whatever the reason, it is not the talking that hits the brakes, it's *your ideas about talking.* Talking can be hot as hell. But the sex imperatives apparently want you to believe that speaking your pleasure or desire, asking for guidance or permission, is anti-pleasure. It's supposed to be effortless. You're supposed to just *know.* You shouldn't have to say it. And if it's not easy, if you do have to talk, everything is ruined.

Go back to my experience with Coen, which I describe in chapter 2. I stopped him, we had to talk about it. The spontaneous desire disappeared in a puff of vapor. And *we still shared a lot of pleasure*. Are you letting the desire imperative stand between you and the pleasure you could experience if you weren't clinging to the need for "spontaneity"?

5. But, Emily, scheduling is so *unromantic* and *unerotic*. I don't care what you say, I want my partner to want me so much they can't help themselves!
Feel free not to schedule sex, if that's not the context that makes pleasure easier to access in your relationship!

I'll take this opportunity to repeat that desire really isn't the thing; pleasure is the thing. Put pleasure at the center of your definition of sexual well-being, and all the other pieces will fall into place.

And yet we know that being wanted is among the most common things people want when they want sex. If you want your partner to want you so much they can't help themselves, and your partner wants to want you so much they can't help themselves, collaborate to create a context that makes that easier—increase things that activate their accelerator and, even more important, decrease things that hit their brakes (see chapter 1 here or, for a lot of detail, see chapter 2 of *Come as You Are* and *The Come as You Are Workbook*).

I also suggest you consider a new version of the questions from chapter 1. Ask yourself, "What is it that I want, when I want my partner to want me so much they can't help themselves?" This can be a difficult question, because it requires acknowledging that you want some pretty vulnerable things. Maybe you want to know that your partner wants all of you, including the parts of yourself you find difficult to accept in yourself—and I bet you can get that in a great relationship. Maybe you want to feel that you are so lovable, so fuckable, that nothing life brings can affect your partner's attraction . . . and I'm not sure that's something many partners can deliver; life hits the brakes for a lot of us, no matter how lovable and fuckable we find our partners. Being wanted is a core need, related to our need for authentic connection. What other experiences, apart from spontaneous desire, fulfill your need to feel fully, deeply welcome, as your whole self, in your erotic relationship?

You'll notice that I am not offering an approach that requires no effort. We don't sustain passionate, spontaneous sexual desire over the long term; we can only re-create it, again and again. And what works to re-create desire will very often be different from what worked last time. Like, remember the movie *Groundhog Day*, where Bill Murray is doomed to live the same day over and over? And one time it goes amazingly, so he tries to re-create that same day, doing the same things, trying to force something that happened organically the first time? You can't force it. You can only create a context that makes it easier.

Important caveat: That's only if your partner also wants to want you that way. If they are *not* interested in wanting you that way, then the conversation is "What is it that I want when I want my partner to want me?" and "What do you not want when you don't want to want me that way?"

6. But I shouldn't have to do all this *work* to make my sex life what it's supposed to be, Emily! You're supposed to be making it easier, not more difficult! Do better!

Yeah, that's a thing we've all been taught, right? That sex is just supposed to happen, easily, no matter what else we have going on in our lives? I hate to be the one to break it to you, but that is not and never was how it works. Sex depends on pleasure; pleasure depends on the context; and the context . . . is not always in our control. I 100 percent own that my advice is much more complicated than "try handcuffs" or even "schedule sex." You are right. I get mad about it, too, sometimes. Why can't it be easier?

I recommend the positive reframe: It's not "difficult" or "work," it's a hobby! It's a mutual interest on which you and your partner collaborate, because you both like it. And if you don't both like it . . . well, the problem isn't that it's so difficult, it's that it's not enjoyable enough to be worth the effort. Fix the pleasure, and the rest will follow.

If you're finding it difficult to be motivated because "it's not supposed to be this effortful," I recommend chapter 2 of *Burnout,* which is about assessing both our goals and the amount of effort we think they're supposed to require. Often, we get frustrated because something takes much more work than we believe it's supposed to, but actually that's just how much work it takes, and if we stop judging how much work it is, we feel more motivated and hopeful and able to notice our progress.

Nobody ever said it would be easy. I would say, though, that it can definitely be worth it.

7. Okay, Emily, but what if I follow your advice and ask my partner to try something new? I started the conversation gently and requested they take their time and respond as nonjudgmentally as they can but my partner not only says no, they *judge* me, thus fulfilling my worst nightmares. Where's your brain science for *that*, huh?

I don't have any brain science for it, but it is an important question!

You have a lot of options, in that moment. You could of course never speak to the person again, pack all your things in the dead of night, move a thousand miles away, and change your identity.

I'm mostly kidding about that, but what if your "something new" is "I'm trans" or "I'm queer" or "I'm kinky and feel most fulfilled as a person when I regularly spend time in sub or dom space"? And what if your partner's reaction is not just a reaction in the moment but a deeply rooted moral judgment? What if you told your person *who you are* and they said, "Nope"?

In a conversation like that, know ahead of time that the stakes may be relationship-endingly high. Talk to a queer/kink/trans-competent therapist in advance. Approach your partner with confidence—knowing what's true—and joy—loving what's true. Do not trade your true self for someone else's approval. Refer to "What You Need," in chapter 10: You need to be who you truly are *and* to be welcomed in a loving community. Maybe you've already spent years sacrificing who you are in order to feel welcome. When you began this conversation with your partner, you were seeking to create that context where all of who you are is welcome. Maybe your partner will need spacious time to process. Maybe your partner can't. There are people who will love all of you, and you deserve to find those people.

But a lot of the things we bring to our partner are not about our identities but our curiosities, interests, pleasures, and questions. The stakes aren't as high. Your partner's unwelcoming reaction to that kind of "something new" could still be about more than the specific thing you're asking about. It might be about a history in your relationship of them going along with what you wanted even when they were ambivalent, but now they're finally speaking up. It might be about your partner's individual history with the specific thing you're discussing or with things they've been taught to feel and believe about different sexual experiences. And while I want to say "explore your partner's response with them, with calm, warm curiosity," I know full well that it's going to be really tough to be there for your partner, when you're hurting from their reaction.

Back to basics: The process of dealing with the feelings caused by a problem is separate from the process of dealing with the problem itself. In this moment, both of you have a ton of difficult feelings. Difficult feelings can hurt, even physically hurt, but they hurt a little less when you can love them as well as you love the most comfortable parts of each other.

Easier said than done, I know. Which is why I explain how to do it with a deliberately silly metaphor in *Come as You Are:*

Imagine that each difficult feeling you experience is a sleepy little hedgehog that you find snoozing in the middle of your favorite chair. You can't relax until you deal with this unexpected visitor.

Find out its name. Its name is likely to be similar to one of the primary process emotions I mentioned in chapter 3. Loneliness. Sadness. Anger. Worry.

Find out what it needs. It might have a specific story, maybe about feeling betrayed or about being exhausted and needing more help. Ultimately what it longs for is to be set free to go live in its true home: a hedge outside your emotional life. Alas, you can't just pick it up and drop it outside your door, you have to help it get what it came for when it wandered into your mental home in the first place.

To find out what it needs, you have to listen to it with—ugh, I know, sorry—kindness and compassion. Also: patience and curiosity.

Also: therapy. These conversations are difficult. You're allowed to recruit some expert help.

8. But, Emily, the desire imperative is just so deeply embedded in my brain; how will I ever stop beating myself up for my responsive desire?

Yeah. You might never be 100 percent done worrying about desire. It's the cycle of woundedness to healing. You're always moving through it. The desire imperative had a long time to entrench itself in your brain, carving a deep, wide wound in your sexual garden. It will take many experiences of feeling free from the desire imperative and then feeling broken again and then feeling liberated again and then feeling ashamed again, but gradually the phases of feeling broken or ashamed will shorten and ease, and the phases of feeling normal, confident, and joyful will expand to fill more and more of your days.

It's not about never feeling broken. It's about welcoming feeling broken as an opportunity to practice remembering that you are not and never were broken.

9. I get that it's important to be patient and meet my partner where they are and whatever, but, Emily, how long am I supposed to wait and be patient before I just give it up as hopeless?

The question here ultimately is "How do I know when to quit?" which is a bigger kind of question than a book about sex can answer. Fortunately, Amelia and I do answer it in chapter 2 of *Burnout*. There's a mechanism we call "the monitor," and understanding how it works will help you know how to tell if you've crossed your threshold and need to stop investing time and energy in something. Then, if you decide to quit, the question becomes more complex. What precisely are you quitting? The whole relationship? The possibility of any sexual connection? And for how long? Are you taking a break?

Or is this a permanent change? You are allowed to stop trying, if trying no longer has any hope of resulting in the change you need.

(Also, really do go read chapter 2 of *Burnout,* because it has some important details about understanding what your goal is and assessing if that goal is actually right for you, and about changing your brain's opinion about how difficult a given goal is supposed to be, aka "criterion velocity." Some goals are much more effortful than we've ever been told.)

10. But, Emily, it's actually true that my partner is the problem. I've tried everything. They refuse to change—they're not even willing to consider change. They won't treat our shared context as a third thing that we turn toward with mutual curiosity. They think I should just shut up and suck it up.
Okay. I've offered a lot of options for what to do when you'd like to create change with a partner or when you want to address old hurts or when you want to understand their experience more clearly or express your experience more clearly. If you have approached your partner with confidence and joy, with calm, warm curiosity, and they are unwilling to reciprocate, maybe your partner truly is the problem—and there certainly are times when they are, in particular when they're deeply in the thrall of the gender mirage, for example. Not all relationships can be saved. Not all relationships are worth saving.

APPENDIX 2

"Because: Biology"

Although the mere existence of transgender, nonbinary, agender, gender-fluid, and other gender-diverse people is, in itself, all the evidence we need that gender is not binary, some people really struggle to accept that not everyone's internal experience of gender is directly tied to the shape of their genitals. If you or someone you know is struggling in this way, I hope this helps.

It's true that when we discuss humans as a species, we are discussing a sexually dimorphic species, meaning we have some individuals with anatomy constructed to produce a large number of extremely small gametes and other individuals with anatomy constructed to produce a limited number of huge gametes. But this population-level description is not accurate as an individual-level description.

That is, just because something is a true statement about the population—e.g., "a sexually dimorphic species"—doesn't mean it's true about every single one of the individuals within that population.

As it happens, there are lots of binaries we impose on bodies and sexuality, beyond gender identity, that aren't *really* binaries, when we look more closely.

Take chromosomes: The usual story we tell is that an ovum slurps up a sperm with a Y sex chromosome or an X sex chromosome. This is where we get chromosomal sex. Let's call "XY" chromosomally male and "XX" chromosomally female. But there are a variety of other combinations of sex chromosomes, like XXY, which is Klinefelter's; XYY, which is creatively called XYY syndrome; or just X with a missing or partially missing second X—that's called Turner's. And none of these are a person's identity; it's literally just their chromosomes. And chromosomes are nonbinary.

How about anatomy? I already mentioned intersex folks, whose genitals are not obviously "It's a girl! or "It's a boy!" shaped when they're born; they're evidence that anatomical sex is also not binary. As with chromosomes, the usual story we tell is that XX fetuses develop external genitalia that adults, seeing them on the newborn baby, will call "girl," and XY fetuses will develop external genitalia that adults will call "boy." In general, the "girl" genitals mean that the urethra is separate from the phallus (clitoris, in this case), and the "boy" genitals mean that the urethra is somewhere on the glans of the phallus (penis, in this case). But some people with XY chromosomes have hypospadias, where the opening of the urethra is somewhere on the shaft of the phallus rather than on the glans. And in congenital adrenal hyperplasia or CAH, a person with XX chromosomes might have a vagina and urethra that converge and open from the body somewhere close to the clitoris, which might be on the larger end of the spectrum and look a lot like a penis. Both intersex conditions are caused by genetic variations that are not the sex chromosomes. Like chromosomes, human genitals are nonbinary. (And again, the shape of someone's genitals doesn't determine their identity; only the person's internal experience determines their identity.)

There are other biological aspects of the thing we call "sex"—

gonadal sex and hormonal sex, for example—and none of them are actually just two options. There's no level of analysis within the body, where "biological sex" is genuinely just two.

Yet, for complicated reasons with deep historical roots, we grow up learning that it's only XX and XY, only vulvas and penises, only girls and boys. I consider it part of the gender mirage that we're taught about just two chromosomal possibilities and not any others. We are taught to see our biology from a point of view that creates a mirage—something you can definitely see but isn't really there. Often, it disappears once you shift your point of view by learning how diverse "biological sex" really is.

I get angry sometimes when I think about how we're lied to about this stuff. It leads intelligent, compassionate people to be wildly confused when they think about people whose gender identities don't match their anatomically assigned role. They say, "There's just two!" because they were never taught that, in fact, there are not just two. There are many levels that a human has a "sex," and not one of them is actually "just two."

So. Biology exists and none of it is binary when it comes to sex. Human psychology (inextricable from human biology) also exists, and none of it is binary, when it comes to gender identity. Culture (inextricable from psychology) exists, too, and we know from the various cultures with other gender categories that these, too, are not binary. It's all a mirage shimmering over the reality of expansive human diversity.

Alfred Kinsey, groundbreaking mid-century sex researcher, began his career as a biologist. He was the world's leading expert on the gall wasp, publishing a five-hundred-page treatise on the topic in 1930. I return to him for inspiration, again and again, for the crucial precision with which he wrote about the nature of intraspecies variety.

> *We may begin our analysis of species by an examination of a few individuals taken in the field. We then become impressed with the truth of the assertion that no two individuals are exactly alike. And if we extend our investigations to*

several dozen individuals, we shall be confused by the vary-
ing characters that enter into any population which ordi-
narily passes as a species. But if, on the other hand, we extend
our examination to several hundred such individuals, we
shall become impressed with another opinion, namely that
there are many more points of uniformity than of varia-
tions among individuals. . . .[1]

It is based on his work that I began teaching one of my central messages: that all of us are made of the same parts, organized in different ways. We are all the same. We are all different. No two alike. That's normal.

ACKNOWLEDGMENTS

Writing a book is, as Amy Poehler puts it, "terrible." It gets done not because I sit in splendid isolation at my keyboard, allowing genius to flow, but because I have long conversations and welcome critical feedback from people I admire. It also gets done because a lot of people help keep my day-to-day life functioning, while I forget to eat or bathe.

This is the page where I get to say thank you to all of them.

Gratitude to the beta readers who read early drafts and offered invaluable feedback about what was helpful and what could go: Steph Auteri, Stephanie Ellis, Kelsey Peterson, Kitty May, Grace, Erika Moen, Sara Nasserzadeh, Chessa Grasso Hickox, Karen Rayne, Elise Clark, Ellice Gonzalez, Elizabeth Goodstein, Kat Stark, Hannah Marcus, Lucie Fielding, Nadine Thornhill, Jaclyn Friedman, Heather Corinna, and many others who preferred to stay anonymous, not to mention literally thousands of newsletter subscribers who responded so thoughtfully to surveys and questions.

And there are my teachers, whose books changed this book. Everyone reading this book, go read their books, too: adrienne maree brown, Andrew Garza, Julian B. Carter, Kai Cheng Thom, Lucie Fielding, Peggy Kleinplatz, Saidiya Hartman, Sebene Selassie, Sue Johnson, and Tricia Hersey.

Also:

My friend, Anna Clutterbuck-Cook.

My sister, Amelia.

My literary agent, Lindsay Edgecombe.

My editor, Sara Weiss.

And last but most, my illustrator and marital euphemism, r stevens. I love you.

NOTES

Introduction: "How Do I Fix It?"

1. Except, perhaps, insofar as people have *expectations* about frequency, and if those expectations are met, people are more satisfied. But aren't we all more satisfied when any of our expectations are met than when they aren't? See Anthony Smith, et al., "Sexual and Relationship Satisfaction Among Heterosexual Men and Women: The Importance of Desired Frequency of Sex," *Journal of Sex & Marital Therapy* 37 (2), (2011): 104–15, and Elizabeth A. Schoenfeld, et al., "Does Sex Really Matter? Examining the Connections Between Spouses' Nonsexual Behaviors, Sexual Frequency, Sexual Satisfaction, and Marital Satisfaction," *Archives of Sexual Behavior* 46 (2), (2017): 489–501.

2. Anik Debrot, et al., "More Than Just Sex: Affection Mediates the Association Between Sexual Activity and Well-being," *Personality and Social Psychology Bulletin* 43 (3), (2017): 287–99; Amy Muise, Elaine Giang, and Emily A. Impett, "Post Sex Affectionate Exchanges Promote Sexual and Relationship Satisfaction," *Archives of Sexual Behavior* 43 (7), (2014): 1391–1402.

3. Among these alternatives, mutual agreement or consent is the theme that unites them all. See Aleta Baldwin, et al., "Sexual Satisfaction in Monoga-

mous, Nonmonogamous, and Unpartnered Sexual Minority Women in the US," *Journal of Bisexuality* 19 (1), (2019): 103–19; Rhonda N. Balzarini and Amy Muise, "Beyond the Dyad: A Review of the Novel Insights Gained from Studying Consensual Non-monogamy," *Current Sexual Health Reports* 12 (4), (2020): 398–404; Terri D. Conley and Jennifer L. Piemonte, "Are There 'Better' and 'Worse' Ways to Be Consensually Non-monogamous (CNM)?: CNM Types and CNM-Specific Predictors of Dyadic Adjustment," *Archives of Sexual Behavior* 50 (4), (2021): 1273–86; Jeffrey T. Parsons, et al., "Non-monogamy and Sexual Relationship Quality Among Same-Sex Male Couples," *Journal of Family Psychology* 26 (5), (2012): 669; Jenna Marie Strizzi et al., "BDSM: Does It Hurt or Help Sexual Satisfaction, Relationship Satisfaction, and Relationship Closeness?" *The Journal of Sex Research,* 59 (2), (2022): 248–57.

4. Peggy Kleinplatz and A. Dana Ménard, *Magnificent Sex: Lessons from Extraordinary Lovers* (Routledge, 2020).

5. "The Fat Spectrum," as illustrated on a widely shared internet graphic originating on *The Fat Lip* podcast, includes "small fats," "mid-fats," "large fats," "superfats," etc. The purpose of the spectrum is not to let us all figure out which kind of fat we are, but to help identify to what extent we might benefit from thin privilege, even when we live in larger bodies. These terms have nothing to do with how we feel—straight-size and midsize people may feel just as self-critical about their bodies as fat people might, and larger people may feel better about their bodies than small people if they've gone further in liberating their inner critic from the Bikini Industrial Complex.

The terms refer instead to *access*. Does your doctor comment on your weight or blame your weight for health issues, or even require you to lose weight before you can have access to a medical treatment? Do your friends or family express "concern" about your body? Can you find clothes that fit you in brick-and-mortar stores? Do seats on public transportation fit your body? These and more are cues about whether your body "belongs" in a culture, regardless of how you feel about that body. As a small fat, I retain some thin privilege (or, "closer proximity to thinness") and have a responsibility not to speak over larger fats who experience more and different oppression (e.g., less access) than I do. For more, see Midnight and Airborne, 2020. "Community Origins of the Term 'Superfat.'" Medium, December 2. Accessed on May 24, 2023. cherrymax.medium.com/community-origins-of -the-term-superfat-9e98e1b0f201; Fluffy Kitten Party, 2021. "Fategories— Understanding the Fat Spectrum." Accessed May 24, 2023. fluffykittenparty .com/2021/06/01/fategories-understanding-smallfat-fragility-the-fat -spectrum/; and Michelle Scott. 2019. "Fat Privilege: Revelations of a Medium Fat Regarding the Fat Spectrum." Medium, August 14. Accessed May 24, 2023. medium.com/@michellevscott/fat-privilege-revelations-of-a -medium-fat-regarding-the-fat-spectrum-ec70dc908336.

Chapter 1: Is Sex Important?

1. Anders Ågmo and Ellen Laan, "The Sexual Incentive Motivation Model and Its Clinical Applications," *The Journal of Sex Research:* 1–20 (2022); Frank A. Beach, "Characteristics of Masculine 'Sex Drive,'" *Nebraska Symposium on Motivation* 4 (1), (1956): 32; and Barry Singer and Frederick M. Toates, "Sexual Motivation," *The Journal of Sex Research* 23 (4), (1987): 481–501. See also *Come as You Are,* chapter 7.

2. If you've never had an orgasm but would like to, there are several books specifically about that, which go far beyond Appendix 1 of *Come as You Are.* I'm also including more general books specifically for survivors of sexual trauma and for trans and nonbinary folks. Any book is a product of its time, and these will show the era in which they were written. See Lonnie Garfield Barbach, *For Yourself: The Fulfillment of Female Sexuality* (Signet, 1976); Vivienne Cass, *The Elusive Orgasm: A Woman's Guide to Why She Can't and How She Can Orgasm* (Brightfire Press, 2002); Betty Dodson, *Sex for One: The Joy of Selfloving* (New York: Harmony Books, 1987); Lucie Fielding, *Trans Sex: Clinical Approaches to Trans Sexualities and Erotic Embodiments* (Routledge, 2021); J. R. Heiman and J. LoPiccolo, *Becoming Orgasmic: A Sexual and Personal Growth Program for Women* (Prentice Hall, 1988); August McLaughlin and Jamila Dawson, *With Pleasure: Managing Trauma Triggers for More Vibrant Sex and Relationships* (Chicago: Chicago Review Press, 2021); Holly Richmond, *Reclaiming Pleasure: A Sex Positive Guide for Moving Past Sexual Trauma and Living a Passionate Life* (New Harbinger Publications, 2021).

3. Don't mistake these answers for science, they're just the responses of a bunch of strangers, mostly on the internet, who happen to follow my work. I didn't keep track of anyone's demographics, I don't know the gender, race, religion, age, sexual orientation, or relationship status of any of the people I quote here, but none of that matters. If someone's words resonate with you, it's not important who the writer is. Same if something doesn't resonate. I'm sharing what I heard from them to help get your brain started on answering this question.

4. Ace sex educator Aubri Lancaster teaches this in her workshops. Hat tip to her! www.AceSexEducation.com.

Chapter 2: Center Pleasure

1. I take this language of "imperatives" from Barker et al., *Mediated Intimacy: Sex Advice in Media Culture.* More on this in chapter 10.

2. Peggy Kleinplatz and A. Dana Ménard, *Magnificent Sex: Lessons from Extraordinary Lovers* (Routledge, 2020); Barry McCarthy and Emily McCarthy, *Contemporary Male Sexuality: Confronting Myths and Promoting Change*

(Routledge, 2020); Jane Fleishman, *The Stonewall Generation: LGBTQ Elders on Sex, Activism, and Aging* (Skinner House Books, 2020).

3. Dear fellow nerds, yes indeed, there's a huge difference between the subjective experience of pleasure and the neurological process of hedonic impact, as there is between the subjective experience of desire and the neurological process of incentive salience. If you know what the difference is, rest assured that I know, too, but this distinction between pleasure and desire is already really difficult for people to wrap their heads around, without going into a discussion of interactions across levels of analysis, and I've found that teaching about levels of analysis doesn't help people have better sex lives, which is the purpose of this book. The science is functioning here as a metaphor. This is one of many, many shortcuts I take in the name of helping people have better sex lives. Feel free to be frustrated by it, if you like, and then remind yourself that you're reading this book to make your sex life better, and this metaphor helps with that. And hey, look up Kent Berridge if you want the science itself!

4. When researchers measure "repair" attempts that couples make to recover trust and positive emotion during a conflict, women's repair attempts are often the most effective. See John M. Gottman, *The Science of Trust: Emotional Attunement for Couples* (New York: W. W. Norton & Company, 2011), 274–9.

5. *Science of Trust,* chapter 7.

6. Donald Hall, "The Third Thing," *Poetry* 185 (2), (2004): 113–21. Hat tip to John Green, *The Anthropocene Reviewed: Essays on a Human-Centered Planet* (Penguin, 2023), for pointing readers to this essay.

7. Kleinplatz and Ménard, *Magnificent Sex.*

Chapter 3: Your Emotional Floorplan

1. I borrow the term "favorable" from the Ace community, where some people identify as "sex favorable," meaning there are some contexts where sex might be fun, even in the absence of sexual attraction that very broadly describes the Ace experience. They use it instead of "sex positive," which already has a variety of connotations in the world. I use favorable instead of "positive," in acknowledgment that many of us have been taught to have negative "secondary emotions" about these primary emotions; that is, we feel self-critical, shameful, fearful, or angry about these "positive" feelings. And I use "adverse" instead of "unfavorable" to underscore that PANIC/GRIEF, FEAR, and RAGE are hardwired to make us motivated to avoid them.

2. Caveat: The book I refer to here is not a book for people looking for science about human sexuality itself; it's about mammals, and a lot of what science can say about mammals, it can't say about humans. See Jaak Panksepp and Lucy Biven, *The Archaeology of Mind: Neuroevolutionary Origins of Human Emotion* (New York: W. W. Norton & Company, 2012).

3. Maybe you prefer to think of these primary process emotions as characters in our personalities; John Gottman offered that type of metaphor to understanding these core emotional systems in his 2001 book, *The Relationship Cure*. He gave each a name and a task: the Jester, the Nest-Builder, the Explorer, etc. You can do the same, thinking about which character moves to the forefront of your mental state as your context changes.

   Or maybe each space is a color, and you can identify where you are by the color that feels right. Or maybe each space is a song that evokes a particular emotion.

   Or maybe you feel most comfortable with the more literal language of primary process emotions being activated as neural networks. Super! Map out the activation and the processes of transitioning from one to another, and the process of activating more than one network at a time. Nan Wise went into detail in her 2020 book, *Why Good Sex Matters*. And if you want to know even more thoroughly what the science already has to say about it, *The Archaeology of Mind* by Jaak Panksepp and Lucy Biven is a detailed place to start.

4. John M. Gottman and Joan DeClaire, *The Relationship Cure: A 5 Step Guide to Strengthening Your Marriage, Family, and Friendships* (Harmony, 2001); Nan Wise, *Why Good Sex Matters: Understanding the Neuroscience of Pleasure for a Smarter, Happier, and More Purpose-Filled Life* (Houghton Mifflin, 2020).

5. Shame, in this framework, is a secondary process emotion, whereas LUST, etc. are primary process emotions. Shame is secondary insofar as it is a *learned response* to social conditioning. See Panksepp and Biven, *Archaeology of Mind*, 10.

6. Barry McCarthy and Emily McCarthy, *Couple Sexuality After 60: Intimate, Pleasurable, and Satisfying* (Routledge, 2021).

7. C. D. Lynch, "How Long Does It Take the Average Couple to Get Pregnant? A Systematic Review of What We Know," *Fertility and Sterility* 96 (3), (2011): S115.

8. "Jealousy Is My Kink," *Dear Jessamyn*, podcast episode 210, originally aired July 2021. Accessed May 24, 2023. dearjessamyn.com/episode-210.

9. Also, they ruin Charlotte. Worst adaptation ever.

10. Amit Bernstein, Yuval Hadash, and David M. Fresco, "Metacognitive Processes Model of Decentering: Emerging Methods and Insights," *Current Opinion in Psychology* 28, (2019): 245–51; Steven C. Hayes, *A Liberated Mind: How to Pivot Toward What Matters* (Penguin, 2020); Richard C. Schwartz, *No Bad Parts: Healing Trauma and Restoring Wholeness with the Internal Family Systems Model* (Sounds True, 2021).

11. Laura Schmalzl and Catherine E. Kerr, "Neural Mechanisms Underlying Movement-Based Embodied Contemplative Practices," *Frontiers in Human Neuroscience* 10, (2016): 169.

Chapter 5: How We Give and Receive

1. When I ask sex-positive providers where to send people who are looking for help with painful sex, they tell me the Herman & Wallace Pelvic Rehabilitation Institute.

Chapter 6: What We Give and Receive

1. Sara Nasserzadeh, *Love by Design: 6 Ingredients to Build a Lifetime of Love* (Balance, 2024).

2. Terrence Real, *Us: Getting Past You and Me to Build a More Loving Relationship* (Rodale Books, 2022).

3. Michael H. Boyle et al., "Differential-Maternal Parenting Behavior: Estimating Within- and Between-Family Effects on Children," *Child Development* 75 (5), (2004): 1457–76; Edward Tronick, et al., "The Infant's Response to Entrapment Between Contradictory Messages in Face-to-Face Interaction," *Journal of the American Academy of Child Psychiatry* 17 (1), (1978): 1–13.

4. Lynne Murray, "Emotional Regulations of Interactions Between Two-Month-Olds and Their Mothers," *Social Perception in Infants* (1985): 177–97.

5. Gottman, *The Science of Trust*, 67.

6. Ibid., 74.

7. I've been waiting for a great adult-focused book about the science of temperament, but so far the book I feel most comfortable recommending is a parenting book. But, as I said to the internship supervisor who recommended it to me, "*I'm* the parent of a spirited child," meaning I have to teach myself to plan for success, given my temperament. See Mary Sheedy Kurcinka, *Raising Your Spirited Child: A Guide for Parents Whose Child Is More Intense, Sensitive, Perceptive, Persistent, and Energetic* (HarperCollins, 2015).

8. Gottman, *The Science of Trust*; Sue Johnson, *Hold Me Tight: Seven Conversations for a Lifetime of Love* (Little, Brown Spark, 2008); David Richo, *How to Be an Adult: A Handbook on Psychological and Spiritual Integration* (Paulist Press, 1991); Richard C. Schwartz, *No Bad Parts: Healing Trauma and Restoring Wholeness with the Internal Family Systems Model* (Sounds True, 2021); Mark Wolynn, *It Didn't Start with You: How Inherited Family Trauma Shapes Who We Are and How to End the Cycle* (Penguin, 2017).

Chapter 7: Living in Bodies

1. Squirmy and Grubs, "Intimacy & Disability—How We Make It Work—Q&A Part 1." YouTube, May 20, 2022. youtube.com/watch?v=8iBROcohmxk; Squirmy and Grubs, "Does Shane's Disease Affect His Sex Drive?—Intimacy and Disability Q&A Part 3." YouTube, June 22, 2020. youtube.com/watch?v =3LJJnULUyFY.

2. StyleLikeU, "Laughing at Your Ableist BS: Shane & Hannah Burcaw Hold a Mirror Up to Your Limited Idea of Love." YouTube, January 20, 2022. youtube.com/watch?v=Y-T39djpGRo&ab_channel=StyleLikeU.

3. Jessica Kellgren-Fozard, "My wife is not an angel// Part I [CC]." YouTube, May 2, 2020. youtube.com/watch?v=-s9GaEha2Nw; Jessica Kellgren-Fozard, "Are there benefits to dating a disabled person?// Part 2: My wife is not an angel [CC]." YouTube, May 5, 2020. youtube.com/watch?v=qUxdPIMTCB8.

4. Staci Haines, *Healing Sex: A Mind-Body Approach to Healing Sexual Trauma* (Cleis Press Start, 2007); August McLaughlin and Jamila Dawson, *With Pleasure: Managing Trauma Triggers for More Vibrant Sex and Relationships* (Chicago: Chicago Review Press, 2021); Holly Richmond, *Reclaiming Pleasure: A Sex Positive Guide for Moving Past Sexual Trauma and Living a Passionate Life* (New Harbinger Publications, 2021); Erika Shershun, *Healing Sexual Trauma Workbook: Somatic Skills to Help You Feel Safe in Your Body, Create Boundaries, and Live with Resilience* (New Harbinger Publications, 2021); David A. Treleaven, *Trauma-Sensitive Mindfulness: Practices for Safe and Transformative Healing* (New York: W. W. Norton & Company, 2018); Bessel A. Van der Kolk, *The Body Keeps the Score: Brain, Mind, and Body in the Healing of Trauma* (Penguin Books, 2015).

Chapter 8: Relationship Change

1. This is a brief description of the Transtheoretical Model or Stages of Change Theory, with Motivational Interviewing applied to the stages. Welcome to the first semester of a Masters in Public Health degree! See Stephen Rollnick, *Motivational Interviewing: Preparing People for Change* (Guilford Press, 2002); James O. Prochaska, "Transtheoretical Model of Behavior Change," *Encyclopedia of Behavioral Medicine,* (2020): 2266–70; James O. Prochaska and W. F. Velicer, "The Transtheoretical Model of Health Behavior Change," *American Journal of Health Promotion* 12 (1), (1997).

2. Any theoretical model that proposes "stages" isn't actually suggesting that people literally shift from one distinct stage to the next, they're simply offering a framework to help contextualize and operationalize the vague and contradictory mess that is real human behavior. There's no need to get too hung up on what exact stage a person is in, we are all in process all the time.

3. Then there's *Relapse,* which is built in to any addiction treatment, normalizing it so that people don't panic if it happens. It applies to changing your shared sexual connection, too, since it's common for people to learn about sex, apply what they've learned, and then, when the going gets tough, revert to old patterns. This isn't a problem, it's a normal part of the process. At this stage, as at all the stages, deploy admiration and trust liberally, practice confidence and joy, meet any self-criticism or frustration with the cycle of woundedness to healing, and approach any interest in further change with calm, warm curiosity. You're doing it, you're making it happen.

4. Amelia has graciously allowed me to share this photo of her with the world.
   From the author's collection.

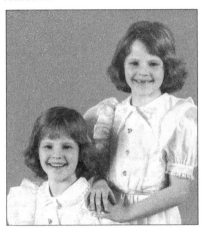

5. Allegra Gordon et al., "Eating Disorders Among Transgender and Gender
   Non-binary People," *Eating Disorders in Boys and Men,* (2021): 265–81.

6. Maria Fernández-Capo, et al., "Measuring Forgiveness: A Systematic Review,"
   European Psychologist 22 (4), (2017): 247.

Chapter 9: The Sex Imperatives

1. Carey Noland, "Communication and Sexual Self-Help: Erotica, Kink and the
   Fifty Shades of Grey Phenomenon," *Sexuality & Culture* 24 (5), (2020):
   1457–79.

2. Book-learning about kink is deeply enriched when you're a part of a community
   that actively practices and teaches safety skills, including consent/communica-
   tion skills. But books are great, too! Here are just a few titles widely recommended in the BDSM community: Molly Devon and Philip Miller, *Screw the
   Roses, Send Me the Thorns: The Romance and Sexual Sorcery of Sadomasochism*
   (Fairfield, CT: Mystic Rose, 1995); Lee Harrington and Mollena Williams, *Playing Well with Others: Your Field Guide to Discovering, Navigating and Exploring
   the Kink, Leather and BDSM Communities* (SCB Distributors, 2012); Tristan
   Taormino, *50 Shades of Kink: An Introduction to BDSM* (Cleis Press, 2012); Jay
   Wiseman, *SM 101: A Realistic Introduction* (CA: Greenery Press, 1996).

3. Jacqueline N. Cohen and E. Sandra Byers, "Beyond Lesbian Bed Death: Enhancing Our Understanding of the Sexuality of Sexual-Minority Women in
   Relationships," *The Journal of Sex Research* 51 (8), (2014): 893–903; Suzanne
   Iasenza, "Beyond 'Lesbian Bed Death' the Passion and Play in Lesbian Relationships," *Journal of Lesbian Studies* 6 (1), (2002): 111–20.

4. Karen L. Blair and Caroline F. Pukall, "Can Less Be More? Comparing Duration vs. Frequency of Sexual Encounters in Same-Sex and Mixed-Sex Relation-

ships," *The Canadian Journal of Human Sexuality* 23 (2), (2014): 123–36; David A. Frederick et al., "Debunking Lesbian Bed Death: Using Coarsened Exact Matching to Compare Sexual Practices and Satisfaction of Lesbian and Heterosexual Women," *Archives of Sexual Behavior* 50 (8), (2021): 3601–19.

5. Karen L. Blair, Jaclyn Cappell, and Caroline F. Pukall, "Not All Orgasms Were Created Equal: Differences in Frequency and Satisfaction of Orgasm Experiences by Sexual Activity in Same-Sex Versus Mixed-Sex Relationships," *The Journal of Sex Research* 55 (6), (2018): 719–33; Jacqueline N. Cohen and E. Sandra Byers, "Beyond Lesbian Bed Death: Enhancing Our Understanding of the Sexuality of Sexual-Minority Women in Relationships," *The Journal of Sex Research* 51 (8), (2014): 893–903; Justin R. Garcia et al., "Variation in Orgasm Occurrence by Sexual Orientation in a Sample of US Singles," *The Journal of Sexual Medicine* 11 (11): 2645–52.

6. Malachi Willis, et al., "Are Women's Orgasms Hindered by Phallocentric Imperatives?" *Archives of Sexual Behavior* 47 (6), (2018): 1565–76.

7. In the time it took me to write this book, hundreds of anti-trans bills were introduced in state legislatures, 63 progressed in the legislature, 73 failed . . . and 98 passed, with more passing each year (20 in 2021; 29 in 2022; and 49 as of this writing in late May 2023). "2023 Anti-Trans Legislation," tracktrans legislation.com/.

YEAR	FAILED	PROGRESSED	PASSED	INTRODUCED
2023 (THROUGH MAY)	29	39	49	413
2022	24	11	29	188
2021	19	13	20	213
TOTAL	73	63	98	814

8. Michele O'Mara, "Lesbian Bed Death Meaning and History," *The Correlation of Sexual Frequency and Relationship Satisfaction Among Lesbians,* 2012. Accessed May 24, 2023. micheleomara.com/lesbian-bed-death-lesbian-sexual-frequency/.

9. American Civil Liberties Union. "Mapping Attacks," Human Rights Watch "LGBT Rights."

10. For details, see chapter 7 of *Come as You Are;* chapter 5 of *Burnout;* Lindo Bacon, *Health at Every Size: The Surprising Truth about Your Weight* (Dallas, TX: BenBella Books, Inc., 2010); and Sonya Renee Taylor, *The Body Is Not an Apology: The Power of Radical Self-love* (Berrett-Koehler Publishers, 2021).

11. Sonalee Rashatwar, "How I Made Peace with My Fat Body and Disappointed My Parents," *Health,* March 19, 2023. Accessed May 24, 2023. health.com

/mind-body/sonalee-rashatwar-how-i-made-peace-with-my-fat-body-health -at-every-size.

12. Diana-Abasi Ibanga, "The Concept of Beauty in African Philosophy," *Africology: The Journal of Pan African Studies* 10 (7): (2017). But also it's complicated, when it comes to gender: see Molly Manyonganise, "Oppressive and Liberative: A Zimbabwean Woman's Reflections on Ubuntu," *Verbum et Ecclesia* 36 (2), (2015): 1–7.

13. Fitz, "The Pieces of the Puzzle," in *Trans Sex: Clinical Approaches to Trans Sexualities and Erotic Embodiments,* ed. Lucie Fielding (Routledge, 2021), 171.

14. Rae McDaniel, *Gender Magic* (Balance, 2023), 113.

Chapter 10: The Gender Mirage

1. I've described a positive scenario, but of course worse situations happen still with alarming frequency, all around the world, as a matter of policy. For example, not until 2020 did Boston Children's Hospital, a leading pediatric care facility, announce that it would not perform *some* intersex surgeries before a patient was old enough to consent. Patient-centered guidelines do exist, and it's long past time that medical practice caught up. See interACT: Advocates for Intersex Youth, Lambda Legal, and Proskauer Rose LLP, 2018, "Intersex-Affirming Hospital Policy Guide: Providing Ethical and Compassionate Health Care to Intersex Patients." legacy.lambdalegal.org/publications/inter sex-affirming.

2. Eustace Chesser, *Love Without Fear: A Plain Guide to Sex Technique for Every Married Adult* (Rich & Cowan, 1941); Betty Friedan, *The Feminine Mystique* (New York: W. W. Norton & Company, 1963); Mike Grace and Joyce Grace, *A Joyful Meeting* (St. Paul, MN: International Marriage Encounter, 1980); Kate Manne, *Down Girl: The Logic of Misogyny* (Oxford University Press, 2017); Barry McCarthy and Emily McCarthy, *Contemporary Male Sexuality: Confronting Myths and Promoting Change* (Routledge, 2020); Jo Barraclough Paoletti, *Pink and Blue: Telling the Boys from the Girls in America* (Indiana University Press, 2012); Sari M. van Anders et al., "The Heteronormativity Theory of Low Sexual Desire in Women Partnered with Men," *Archives of Sexual Behavior* 51 (1), (2022): 391–415.

3. Nagoski and Nagoski, *Burnout,* xiii and 62–65.

4. Ågmo and Laan, "The Sexual Incentive Motivation Model." See also chapter 7 of *Come as You Are.*

5. McCarthy and McCarthy, *Contemporary Male Sexuality.*

6. Yoko Kanemasu and Asenati Liki, "'Let *Fa'afafine* Shine Like Diamonds': Balancing Accommodation, Negotiation and Resistance in Gender-Nonconforming Samoans' Counter-hegemony," *Journal of Sociology* 57 (4), (2021): 806–24.

7. Wesley Thomas, "Navajo Cultural Constructions of Gender and Sexuality," *Two-Spirit People: Native American Gender Identity, Sexuality, and Spirituality,* (1997): 156–73.

8. Sharyn Davies, *Challenging Gender Norms: Five Genders among Bugis in Indonesia* (Gale Cengage, 2007).

9. Oyèrónké Oyěwùmí, *The Invention of Women: Making an African Sense of Western Gender Discourses* (University of Minnesota Press, 1997).

10. Sandy O'Sullivan, "The Colonial Project of Gender (and Everything Else)," *Genealogy* 5 (3), (2021): 67.

11. Joseph M. Currin, et al., "Gender Normative Behavior as a Predictor of Acceptance of Transgender Individuals in the Workplace by Cisgender Coworkers," *Journal of LGBTQ Issues in Counseling* 16 (2), (2022): 169–85.

12. McCarthy and McCarthy, *Couple Sexuality After 60,* 57.

Chapter 11: Heterosexual-Type Relationships

1. Beyond countless online articles about "Top 10 Complaints Wives Have about Their Husbands" and "5 Things Men Can't Stand about Their Wives," not to mention memoirs of marriage, these are also grounded in clinical practice and empirical research. See John M. Gottman, "How Marriages Change," *Depression and Aggression in Family Interaction,* edited by G. R. Patterson (1990): 75–101. Lawrence Erlbaum Associates, Inc.: 89; Heather Havrilesky, *Foreverland: On the Divine Tedium of Marriage* (Ecco, 2022); Harrison Scott Key, *How to Stay Married: The Most Insane Love Story Ever Told* (Avid Reader Press / Simon & Schuster, 2023); Kate Mangino, *Equal Partners: Improving Gender Equality at Home* (St. Martin's Press, 2022); Terrence Real, *How Can I Get Through to You?: Closing the Intimacy Gap Between Men and Women* (Scribner, 2010).

2. In her famous (and eugenicist) sex advice manual, *Married Love,* Marie Stopes includes an entire chapter on "Woman's Contrariness," which she attributes to the menstrual cycle. A century later, we know the link between the menstrual cycle and sexual interest, feelings, and behavior is not remotely this straightforward. See Lisa M. Diamond., et al., "Menstrual Cycle Changes in Daily Sexual Motivation and Behavior Among Sexually Diverse Cisgender Women," *Archives of Sexual Behavior* (2022): 1–12; Urszula M. Marcinkowska, et al., "Hormonal Underpinnings of the Variation in Sexual Desire, Arousal and Activity Throughout the Menstrual Cycle–A Multifaceted Approach," *The Journal of Sex Research* (2022): 1–7; Marie Stopes, *Married Love: A New Contribution to the Solution of Sex Differences* (London: G. Putnam's Sons, 1918); Sari M. van Anders et al., "The Heteronormativity Theory of Low Sexual Desire in Women Partnered with Men," *Archives of Sexual Behavior* 51 (1), (2022): 391–415.

3. Ernest Jones, *The Life and Work of Sigmund Freud, Vol. 1. The formative years and the great discoveries, 1856–1900* (1953).

4. *The American Magazine*, Crowell-Collier Publishing Company, 1911, 619.

5. Editor, "Training for Freedom: We Want Bread—and Roses Too."

6. Saidiya Hartman, *Wayward Lives, Beautiful Experiments: Intimate Histories of Riotous Black Girls, Troublesome Women, and Queer Radicals* (New York: W. W. Norton & Company, 2019).

7. Sigmund Freud, "The Psychical Consequences of the Anatomic Distinction Between the Sexes." *Complete Psychological Works of Sigmund Freud: "The Ego and the Id" and Other Works* 19 (1925) 2014: 242–60.

8. Heidi Staufenberg, "8.6 Female Psychosexuality," *Freud-Handbuch Leben Werk Wirkung Sonderausgabe,* edited by Hans-Martin Lohmann and Joachim Pfeiffer (Stuttgart, Germany: Springer-Verlag, 2006): 162–67.

Chapter 12: The Magic Trick

1. Fred B. Bryant and Joseph Veroff, *Savoring: A New Model of Positive Experience* (Psychology Press, 2017).

2. Ibid., xx. The remaining savoring skills, still applicable to the erotic, but maybe a little less straightforward, include:

- *Memory Building.* Actively choosing positive moments to highlight in your awareness, to store for future reminiscing.

- *Self-congratulation.* Pausing to celebrate privately, to tell yourself how proud you are or how impressed others must be.

- *Comparing.* Contrast your own feelings with what others seem to be feeling, or comparing the present situation with similar times in the past or other potential outcomes. This is the "coulda been so much worse!" strategy.

- *Counting Blessings.* Remind yourself of all the good things you have or experience, even in the midst of other not-so-good things.

- *Absorption.* This is a strategy many might describe with the concept of "flow." Exist only in the present, not worrying about the future or ruminating on the past.

3. Shemeka Thorpe, et al., "The Peak of Pleasure: US Southern Black Women's Definitions of and Feelings Toward Sexual Pleasure," *Sexuality & Culture* 26 (3), (2022): 1115–31; Shemeka Thorpe, et al., "Black Queer Women's Pleasure: A Review," *Current Sexual Health Reports,* (2023): 1–7.

Pleasure Mountain, as Thorpe discovered from her research participants' accounts of sexual pleasure, has three foundational dimensions and four Facilitators of Peak Pleasure.

THE THREE DIMENSIONS:

- The <u>emotional dimension</u> of sexual pleasure is about the experience of emotional closeness and connection to a partner, including euphoric experience of compassion, tenderness, care, and vulnerability. This is the dimension participants described with the word "love."

- The <u>mental dimension</u> of sexual pleasure is about being present, undistracted, and able to "let go." It's like the experience I called Freedom in chapter 1, the feeling of being released from all the other noise happening in their lives, plus a sense that their expectations and desires were satisfied. For this dimension, participants used words like satisfaction, contentment, and delight.

- The <u>physical dimension</u> of sexual pleasure is related to body sensations, particularly—and this is a crucial feature of this dimension—the post-sex, "resolution" phase of the experience. The release of physical tension was as much a part of the experience of sexual pleasure as orgasm itself. This dimension isn't about emotion but about bodily sensations per se, from a whole-body tingling to flushing and heat to genital sensations to the experience of physical release.

THE FOUR FACILITATORS:

- Partnered interactions are about feeling mutual satisfaction or the ability to give pleasure to their partner, for example hearing them moan.

- Liberation is particularly related to the mental dimension of sexual pleasure. About 19 percent of research participants described sexual pleasure as feeling completely uninhibited and unencumbered. This isn't just the Freedom I described in chapter 1, which was really freedom from stress and worries and inhibitions. This experience of liberation was bigger, a kind of full liberation from the "shoulds" of how Black women are supposed to be sexual. That creates a context where they could fully enjoy sexual pleasure on their own terms. And liberation allowed for the experience of sexual agency, particularly the dual experience of both being fully in control and also being free to be out of control.

- Mind-body-soul awareness is similar to Kleinplatz and Ménard's description of participants' ability to be fully present and aware in their own bodies, while also being closely attuned to their partners' bodies.

- Orgasm, whether individual or mutual. Crucially, many participants' descriptions of this facilitator weren't just "having an orgasm," but rather the whole process of growing arousal and pleasure, increasing physical tension, and then the culmination of orgasm. As a facilitator of peak pleasure, orgasm isn't "just" orgasm, it's journeying across your sexual terrain to the land of orgasm.

4. Kleinplatz and Ménard, *Magnificent Sex*.

5. Jess Tarpey, et al., *The Bump'n Book of Love, Lust & Disability*.

Appendix 2: "Because: Biology"

1. Alfred Kinsey, *The Gall Wasp Genus Cynips: A Study in the Origin of Species*, in *Indiana University Studies vol. XVI* (Bloomington, IN: Indiana University, 1930), 18.

REFERENCES

Ågmo, Anders, and Ellen Laan. 2022. "The Sexual Incentive Motivation Model and Its Clinical Applications." *The Journal of Sex Research:* 1–20.

American Civil Liberties Union. "Mapping Attacks on LGBTQ Rights in U.S. State Legislatures." Accessed May 24, 2023. aclu.org/legislative-attacks-on-lgbtq-rights.

Bacon, Lindo. 2010. *Health at Every Size: The Surprising Truth about Your Weight.* Dallas, TX: BenBella Books, Inc.

Baldwin, Aleta, Debby Herbenick, Vanessa R. Schick, Brenda Light, Brian Dodge, Crystal A. Jackson, and J. Dennis Fortenberry. 2019. "Sexual Satisfaction in Monogamous, Nonmonogamous, and Unpartnered Sexual Minority Women in the US." *Journal of Bisexuality* 19 (1): 103–19.

Balzarini, Rhonda N., and Amy Muise. 2020. "Beyond the Dyad: A Review of the Novel Insights Gained from Studying Consensual Non-monogamy." *Current Sexual Health Reports* 12 (4): 398–404.

Barbach, Lonnie Garfield. 1976. *For Yourself: The Fulfillment of Female Sexuality.* Signet.

Beach, Frank A. 1956. "Characteristics of Masculine 'Sex Drive.'" *Nebraska Symposium on Motivation* 4 (1): 32.

Bernstein, Amit, Yuval Hadash, and David M. Fresco. 2019. "Metacognitive Processes Model of Decentering: Emerging Methods and Insights." *Current Opinion in Psychology* 28: 245–51.

Blair, Karen L., Jaclyn Cappell, and Caroline F. Pukall. 2018. "Not All Orgasms Were Created Equal: Differences in Frequency and Satisfaction of Orgasm Experiences by Sexual Activity in Same-Sex Versus Mixed-Sex Relationships." *The Journal of Sex Research* 55 (6): 719–33.

Blair, Karen L., and Caroline F. Pukall. 2014. "Can Less Be More? Comparing Duration vs. Frequency of Sexual Encounters in Same-Sex and Mixed-Sex Relationships." *The Canadian Journal of Human Sexuality* 23 (2): 123–36.

Boyle, Michael H., Jennifer M. Jenkins, Katholiki Georgiades, John Cairney, Eric Duku, and Yvonne Racine. 2004. "Differential-Maternal Parenting Behavior: Estimating Within- and Between-Family Effects on Children." *Child Development* 75 (5): 1457–76.

Bryant, Fred B., and Joseph Veroff. 2017. *Savoring: A New Model of Positive Experience.* Psychology Press.

Cass, Vivienne. 2002. *The Elusive Orgasm: A Woman's Guide to Why She Can't and How She Can Orgasm.* Brightfire Press.

Chesser, Eustace. 1941. *Love Without Fear: A Plain Guide to Sex Technique for Every Married Adult.* Rich & Cowan.

Cohen, Jacqueline N., and E. Sandra Byers. 2014. "Beyond Lesbian Bed Death: Enhancing Our Understanding of the Sexuality of Sexual-Minority Women in Relationships." *The Journal of Sex Research* 51 (8): 893–903.

Conley, Terri D., and Jennifer L. Piemonte. 2021. "Are There 'Better' and 'Worse' Ways to Be Consensually Non-monogamous (CNM)?: CNM Types and CNM-Specific Predictors of Dyadic Adjustment." *Archives of Sexual Behavior* 50 (4): 1273–86.

Currin, Joseph M., Lindsay Rice, Amelia E. Evans, Hannah R. Snidman, and Cameron D. Taylor. 2022. "Gender Normative Behavior as a Predictor of Acceptance of Transgender Individuals in the Workplace by Cisgender Co-workers." *Journal of LGBTQ Issues in Counseling* 16 (2): 169–85.

Davies, Sharyn. 2007. *Challenging Gender Norms: Five Genders among Bugis in Indonesia.* Gale Cengage.

Debrot, Anik, Nathalie Meuwly, Amy Muise, Emily A. Impett, and Dominik Schoebi. 2017. "More Than Just Sex: Affection Mediates the Association Between Sexual Activity and Well-being." *Personality and Social Psychology Bulletin* 43 (3): 287–99.

Devon, Molly, and Philip Miller. 1995. *Screw the Roses, Send Me the Thorns: The Romance and Sexual Sorcery of Sadomasochism.* Fairfield, CT: Mystic Rose.

Diamond, Lisa M., Janna A. Dickenson, and Karen L. Blair. 2022. "Menstrual Cycle Changes in Daily Sexual Motivation and Behavior Among Sexually Diverse Cisgender Women." *Archives of Sexual Behavior:* 1–12.

Dodson, Betty. 1987. *Sex for One: The Joy of Selfloving.* New York: Harmony Books.

Editor. 1918. "Training for Freedom: We Want Bread—and Roses Too." *Life and Labor: A Monthly Magazine* 8: 189.

Fernández-Capo, Maria, Silvia Recoder Fernández, María Gámiz Sanfeliu, Juana Gómez Benito, and Everett L. Worthington Jr. 2017. "Measuring Forgiveness: A Systematic Review." *European Psychologist* 22 (4): 247.

Fielding, Lucie. 2021. *Trans Sex: Clinical Approaches to Trans Sexualities and Erotic Embodiments.* Routledge.

Fleishman, Jane. 2020. "The Stonewall Generation: LGBTQ Elders on Sex, Activism, and Aging." Skinner House Books.

Fluffy Kitten Party. 2021. "Fategories—Understanding the Fat Spectrum." Accessed May 24, 2023. fluffykittenparty.com/2021/06/01/fategories -understanding-smallfat-fragility-the-fat-spectrum/.

Frederick, David A., Brian Joseph Gillespie, Janet Lever, Vincent Berardi, and Justin R. Garcia. 2021. "Debunking Lesbian Bed Death: Using Coarsened Exact Matching to Compare Sexual Practices and Satisfaction of Lesbian and Heterosexual Women." *Archives of Sexual Behavior* 50 (8): 3601–19.

Freud, Sigmund. (1925) 2014. "The Psychical Consequences of the Anatomic Distinction Between the Sexes." *Complete Psychological Works of Sigmund Freud: "The Ego and the Id" and Other Works* 19: 242–60.

Friedan, Betty. 1963. *The Feminine Mystique.* New York: W. W. Norton & Company.

Garcia, Justin R., Elisabeth A. Lloyd, Kim Wallen, and Helen E. Fisher. "Variation in Orgasm Occurrence by Sexual Orientation in a Sample of US Singles." *The Journal of Sexual Medicine* 11 (11): 2645–52.

Gignac, Gilles E., Joey Darbyshire, and Michelle Ooi. 2018. "Some People Are Attracted Sexually to Intelligence: A Psychometric Evaluation of Sapiosexuality." *Intelligence* 66: 98–111.

Gordon, Allegra R., L. B. Moore, and Carly Guss. 2021. "Eating Disorders Among Transgender and Gender Non-binary People." In *Eating Disorders in Boys and Men,* edited by J. M. Nagata et al., 265–81. Springer International Publishing.

Gottman, John M. 1990. "How Marriages Change." In *Depression and Aggression in Family Interaction,* edited by G. R. Patterson, 75–101. Lawrence Erlbaum Associates, Inc.: 89.

———. 2011. *The Science of Trust: Emotional Attunement for Couples.* New York: W. W. Norton & Company.

Gottman, John M., and Joan DeClaire. 2001. *The Relationship Cure: A 5 Step Guide to Strengthening Your Marriage, Family, and Friendships.* Harmony.

Grace, Mike, and Joyce Grace. 1980. "A Joyful Meeting." St. Paul, MN: International Marriage Encounter.

Green, John. 2023. *The Anthropocene Reviewed: Essays on a Human-Centered Planet.* Penguin.

Haines, Staci. 2007. *Healing Sex: A Mind-Body Approach to Healing Sexual Trauma.* Cleis Press Start.

Hall, Donald. 2004. "The Third Thing." *Poetry* 185 (2): 113–21.

Harrington, Lee, and Mollena Williams. 2012. *Playing Well with Others: Your Field Guide to Discovering, Navigating and Exploring the Kink, Leather and BDSM Communities.* SCB Distributors.

Hartman, Saidiya. 2019. *Wayward Lives, Beautiful Experiments: Intimate Histories of Riotous Black Girls, Troublesome Women, and Queer Radicals.* New York: W. W. Norton & Company.

Havrilesky, Heather. 2022. *Foreverland: On the Divine Tedium of Marriage.* Ecco.

Hayes, Steven C. 2020. *A Liberated Mind: How to Pivot Toward What Matters.* Penguin.

Heiman, J. R., and J. LoPiccolo. 1988. *Becoming Orgasmic: A Sexual and Personal Growth Program for Women.* Prentice Hall.

Human Rights Watch. "LGBT Rights." Accessed May 24, 2023. hrw.org/topic/lgbt-rights.

Iasenza, Suzanne. 2002. "Beyond 'Lesbian Bed Death' the Passion and Play in Lesbian Relationships." *Journal of Lesbian Studies* 6 (1): 111–20.

Ibanga, Diana-Abasi. 2017. "The Concept of Beauty in African Philosophy." *Africology: The Journal of Pan African Studies* 10 (7).

interACT: Advocates for Intersex Youth, Lambda Legal, and Proskauer Rose LLP. 2018. "Intersex-Affirming Hospital Policy Guide: Providing Ethical and Compassionate Health Care to Intersex Patients." legacy.lambdalegal.org/publications/intersex-affirming.

Johnson, Sue. 2008. *Hold Me Tight: Seven Conversations for a Lifetime of Love.* Little, Brown Spark.

Kanemasu, Yoko, and Asenati Liki. 2021. "'Let *Fa'afafine* Shine Like Diamonds': Balancing Accommodation, Negotiation and Resistance in Gender-Nonconforming Samoans' Counter-hegemony." *Journal of Sociology* 57 (4): 806–24.

Key, Harrison Scott. 2023. *How to Stay Married: The Most Insane Love Story Ever Told.* Avid Reader Press / Simon & Schuster.

Kleinplatz, Peggy, and A. Dana Ménard. 2020. *Magnificent Sex: Lessons from Extraordinary Lovers.* Routledge.

Kurcinka, Mary Sheedy. 2015. *Raising Your Spirited Child: A Guide for Parents Whose Child Is More Intense, Sensitive, Perceptive, Persistent, and Energetic.* HarperCollins.

Lynch, C. D. 2011. "How Long Does It Take the Average Couple to Get Pregnant? A Systematic Review of What We Know." *Fertility and Sterility* 96 (3): S115.

Mangino, Kate. 2022. *Equal Partners: Improving Gender Equality at Home.* St. Martin's Press.

Manne, Kate. 2017. *Down Girl: The Logic of Misogyny.* Oxford University Press.

Manyonganise, Molly. 2015. "Oppressive and Liberative: A Zimbabwean Woman's Reflections on *Ubuntu.*" *Verbum et Ecclesia* 36 (2): 1–7.

Marcinkowska, Urszula M., Talia Shirazi, Magdalena Mijas, and James R. Roney. 2022. "Hormonal Underpinnings of the Variation in Sexual Desire, Arousal and Activity Throughout the Menstrual Cycle–A Multifaceted Approach." *The Journal of Sex Research:* 1–7.

McCarthy, Barry, and Emily McCarthy. 2020. *Contemporary Male Sexuality: Confronting Myths and Promoting Change.* Routledge.

———. 2021. *Couple Sexuality After 60: Intimate, Pleasurable, and Satisfying.* Routledge.

McDaniel, Rae. 2023. *Gender Magic: Live Shamelessly, Reclaim Your Joy, & Step into Your Most Authentic Self.* Balance.

McLaughlin, August, and Jamila Dawson. 2021. *With Pleasure: Managing Trauma Triggers for More Vibrant Sex and Relationships.* Chicago: Chicago Review Press.

Michael, Darcy, and Jeremy Baer. "Pop Quiz Throwback." YouTube. Accessed on May 24, 2023. youtube.com/shorts/dye9J17UfFg.

Midnight, Cherry, and Max Airborne. 2020. "Community Origins of the Term 'Superfat.'" Medium, December 2. Accessed on May 24, 2023. cherrymax .medium.com/community-origins-of-the-term-superfat-9e98e1b0f201.

Muise, Amy, Elaine Giang, and Emily A. Impett. 2014. "Post Sex Affectionate Exchanges Promote Sexual and Relationship Satisfaction." *Archives of Sexual Behavior* 43 (7): 1391–1402.

Murray, Lynne. 1985. "Emotional Regulations of Interactions Between Two-Month-Olds and Their Mothers." *Social Perception in Infants:* 177–97.

Nasserzadeh, Sara. 2024. *Love by Design: 6 Ingredients to Build a Lifetime of Love.* Balance.

Noland, Carey. 2020. "Communication and Sexual Self-Help: Erotica, Kink and the *Fifty Shades of Grey* Phenomenon." *Sexuality & Culture* 24 (5): 1457–79.

O'Mara, Michele. 2012. "Lesbian Bed Death Meaning and History." *The Correlation of Sexual Frequency and Relationship Satisfaction Among Lesbians.* Accessed May 24, 2023. micheleomara.com/lesbian-bed-death-lesbian-sexual-frequency/.

O'Sullivan, Sandy. 2021. "The Colonial Project of Gender (and Everything Else)." *Genealogy* 5 (3): 67.

Oyěwùmí, Oyèrónkẹ́. 1997. *The Invention of Women: Making an African Sense of Western Gender Discourses.* University of Minnesota Press.

Panksepp, Jaak, and Lucy Biven. 2012. *The Archaeology of Mind: Neuroevolutionary Origins of Human Emotion.* New York: W. W. Norton & Company.

Paoletti, Jo Barraclough. 2012. *Pink and Blue: Telling the Boys from the Girls in America.* Indiana University Press.

Parsons, Jeffrey T., Tyrel J. Starks, Kristi E. Gamarel, and Christian Grov. 2012. "Non-monogamy and Sexual Relationship Quality Among Same-Sex Male Couples." *Journal of Family Psychology* 26 (5): 669.

Prochaska, James O. 2020. "Transtheoretical Model of Behavior Change." In *Encyclopedia of Behavioral Medicine,* 2266–70.

Prochaska, James O., and W. F. Velicer. 1997. "The Transtheoretical Model of Health Behavior Change." *American Journal of Health Promotion* 12 (1).

Rashatwar, Sonalee. 2023. "How I Made Peace with My Fat Body and Disappointed My Parents." *Health,* March 19. Accessed May 24, 2023. health.com/mind-body/sonalee-rashatwar-how-i-made-peace-with-my-fat-body-health-at-every-size.

Real, Terrence. 2010. *How Can I Get Through to You?: Closing the Intimacy Gap Between Men and Women.* Scribner.

———2022. *Us: Getting Past You and Me to Build a More Loving Relationship.* Rodale Books.

Richmond, Holly. 2021. *Reclaiming Pleasure: A Sex Positive Guide for Moving Past Sexual Trauma and Living a Passionate Life.* New Harbinger Publications.

Richo, David. 1991. *How to Be an Adult: A Handbook on Psychological and Spiritual Integration.* Paulist Press.

Rollnick, Stephen. 2002. *Motivational Interviewing: Preparing People for Change*. Guilford Press.

Rumi. (2004). *The Essential Rumi* (New Expanded Edition). Translated by Coleman Barks. San Francisco: HarperOne.

Schmalzl, Laura, and Catherine E. Kerr. 2016. "Neural Mechanisms Underlying Movement-Based Embodied Contemplative Practices." *Frontiers in Human Neuroscience* 10: 169.

Schoenfeld, Elizabeth A., Timothy J. Loving, Mark T. Pope, Ted L. Huston, and Aleksandar Štulhofer. 2017. "Does Sex Really Matter? Examining the Connections Between Spouses' Nonsexual Behaviors, Sexual Frequency, Sexual Satisfaction, and Marital Satisfaction." *Archives of Sexual Behavior* 46 (2): 489–501.

Schwartz, Richard C. 2021. *No Bad Parts: Healing Trauma and Restoring Wholeness with the Internal Family Systems Model*. Sounds True.

Scott, Michelle V. 2019. "Fat Privilege: Revelations of a Medium Fat Regarding the Fat Spectrum." Medium, August 14. Accessed May 24, 2023. medium .com/@michellevscott/fat-privilege-revelations-of-a-medium-fat-regarding -the-fat-spectrum-ec70dc908336.

Shershun, Erika. 2021. *Healing Sexual Trauma Workbook: Somatic Skills to Help You Feel Safe in Your Body, Create Boundaries, and Live with Resilience*. New Harbinger Publications.

Singer, Barry, and Frederick M. Toates. 1987. "Sexual Motivation." *The Journal of Sex Research* 23 (4): 481–501.

Smith, Anthony, Anthony Lyons, Jason Ferris, Juliet Richters, Marian Pitts, Julia Shelley, and Judy M. Simpson. 2011. "Sexual and Relationship Satisfaction Among Heterosexual Men and Women: The Importance of Desired Frequency of Sex." *Journal of Sex & Marital Therapy* 37 (2): 104–15.

Staufenberg, Heidi. 2006. "8.6 Female Psychosexuality." In *Freud-Handbuch Leben Werk Wirkung Sonderausgabe*, edited by Hans-Martin Lohmann and Joachim Pfeiffer, 162–67. Stuttgart, Germany: Springer-Verlag.

Stopes, Marie. 1918. "Married Love: A New Contribution to the Solution of Sex Differences." London: G. Putnam's Sons.

Strizzi, Jenna Marie, Camilla Stine Øverup, Ana Ciprić, Gert Martin Hald, and Bente Træen. 2022. "BDSM: Does It Hurt or Help Sexual Satisfaction, Relationship Satisfaction, and Relationship Closeness?" *The Journal of Sex Research* 59 (2): 248–57.

StyleLikeU. 2022. "Laughing at Your Ableist BS: Shane & Hannah Burcaw Hold a Mirror Up to Your Limited Idea of Love." YouTube, January 20. youtube.com/watch?v=Y-T39djpGRo&ab_channel=StyleLikeU.

Taormino, Tristan. 2012. *50 Shades of Kink: An Introduction to BDSM*. Cleis Press.

Tarpey, Jess, Andrew Gurza, and Katy Venables. *The Bump'n Book of Love, Lust & Disability.* Sydney: getbumpn.com/products/e-book-the-bumpn-book-of-love-lust-disability.

Taylor, Sonya Renee. 2021. *The Body Is Not an Apology: The Power of Radical Self-love.* Berrett-Koehler Publishers.

Thomas, Wesley. 1997. "Navajo Cultural Constructions of Gender and Sexuality." *Two-Spirit People: Native American Gender Identity, Sexuality, and Spirituality:* 156–73.

Thorpe, Shemeka, Natalie Malone, Candice N. Hargons, Jardin N. Dogan, and Jasmine K. Jester. 2022. "The Peak of Pleasure: US Southern Black Women's Definitions of and Feelings Toward Sexual Pleasure." *Sexuality & Culture* 26 (3): 1115–31.

Thorpe, Shemeka, Natalie Malone, Rayven L. Peterson, Praise Iyiewuare, Monyae Kerney, and Candice N. Hargons. 2023. "Black Queer Women's Pleasure: A Review." *Current Sexual Health Reports:* 1–7.

Treleaven, David A. 2018. *Trauma-Sensitive Mindfulness: Practices for Safe and Transformative Healing.* New York: W. W. Norton & Company.

Tronick, Edward, Heidelise Als, Lauren Adamson, Susan Wise, and T. Berry Brazelton. 1978. "The Infant's Response to Entrapment Between Contradictory Messages in Face-to-Face Interaction." *Journal of the American Academy of Child Psychiatry* 17 (1): 1–13.

van Anders, Sari M., Debby Herbenick, Lori A. Brotto, Emily A. Harris, and Sara B. Chadwick. 2022. "The Heteronormativity Theory of Low Sexual Desire in Women Partnered with Men." *Archives of Sexual Behavior* 51 (1): 391–415.

Van der Kolk, Bessel A. 2015. *The Body Keeps the Score: Brain, Mind, and Body in the Healing of Trauma.* Penguin Books.

Willis, Malachi, Kristen N. Jozkowski, Wen-Juo Lo, and Stephanie A. Sanders. 2018. "Are Women's Orgasms Hindered by Phallocentric Imperatives?" *Archives of Sexual Behavior* 47 (6): 1565–76.

Wise, Nan. 2020. *Why Good Sex Matters: Understanding the Neuroscience of Pleasure for a Smarter, Happier, and More Purpose-Filled Life.* Houghton Mifflin.

Wiseman, Jay. 1996. *SM 101: A Realistic Introduction.* CA: Greenery Press.

Wolynn, Mark. 2017. *It Didn't Start with You: How Inherited Family Trauma Shapes Who We Are and How to End the Cycle.* Penguin.

INDEX

ABOUT THE AUTHOR

EMILY NAGOSKI is the *New York Times* bestselling, award-winning author of *Come as You Are* and co-author, with her sister, Amelia, of *Burnout: The Secret to Unlocking the Stress Cycle*. She earned an MS in counseling and a PhD in health behavior, both from Indiana University, with clinical and research training at the Kinsey Institute. Now she combines sex education and stress education to teach women to live with confidence and joy inside their bodies. She lives in Massachusetts with two dogs, a cat, and a cartoonist.